Therapeutic Skills for Mental Health Nurses

Therapeutic Skills for Mental Health Nurses

Edited by Nicola Evans and Ben Hannigan

Mc
Graw
Hill
Education
Open University Press

Open University Press
McGraw-Hill Education
8th Floor
338 Euston Road
London
NW1 3BH

email: enquiries@openup.co.uk
world wide web: www.openup.co.uk

and Two Penn Plaza, New York, NY 10121-2289, USA

First published 2016

A catalogue record of this book is available from the British Library

ISBN-13: 978-0-33-526440-7
ISBN-10: 0-33-526440-9
eISBN: 978-0-33-526441-4

Library of Congress Cataloging-in-Publication Data
CIP data applied for

Typeset by Aptara, Inc.

Fictitious names of companies, products, people, characters and/or data that may be
used herein (in case studies or in examples) are not intended to represent any real
individual, company, product or event.

Printed and bound by CPI Group (UK) Ltd, Croydon, CR0 4YY

Praise page

"Whilst the essential therapeutic component of mental health nursing is the nurse themselves, it is also essential that they have knowledge and competencies to offer the client. This valuable book offers the reader an introduction to a wide range of approaches that are considered helpful, evidence based and effective. Modern mental health nursing requires much of its practitioners; this book will help inform and support that endeavour."

Ian Hulatt, Mental Health Adviser,
Royal College of Nursing, UK

"This is a timely book which addresses, head on, questions about what mental health nurses can do to be effective with their patients. At last we have a book that mental health nurses can draw on to understand why and how various therapeutic approaches are used. The range is from cognitive behavioural therapy, to psychodynamic approaches to mindfulness, with others in between.

Each chapter is written by an expert and each offers concrete examples of what it involved in each of the approaches. These examples are imperative if readers are to understand how to use interventions in their everyday work.

This ground breaking book will be compulsory reading for everyone involved in the care of those with mental health problems. A wonderful book."

Philip Burnard, Emeritus Professor of Nursing,
Cardiff University, UK

Contents

List of editors and contributors   ix

Part 1: Foundations for practice   **1**

    Preface: Introducing therapeutic skills   3
    NICOLA EVANS AND BEN HANNIGAN

1   Conducting assessment interviews   6
    GERWYN JONES AND NORMAN YOUNG

2   Clinical supervision   21
    JESSICA MACLAREN

Part 2: Therapeutic skills   **33**

3   Person-centred counselling   35
    THEO STICKLEY AND PAUL CASSEDY

4   Using a solution-focused approach   49
    NICOLA EVANS

5   Motivational interviewing   60
    MICHELLE HUWS-THOMAS

6   Using the skills of problem solving   74
    STEVEN PRYJMACHUK

7   The skill of offering psychoeducation   88
    JOHN HYDE

8   Skills to challenge unhelpful thoughts   102
    JO SULLIVAN

9   Validation skills applied to people with dementia   117
    PAUL BICKERSTAFFE AND AMANDA KING

10 Preventing relapse 130
IAIN RYRIE

11 Behavioural management and activation 143
GEOFF BRENNAN

12 Mindfulness 154
SALI BURNS AND STEVE RILEY

13 De-escalating volatile situations 167
ELIZABETH BOWRING-LOSSOCK

Part 3: Working with families and groups **179**

14 Working systemically with families in mind 181
BILLY HARDY

15 Working with groups 192
ALEX NUTE

16 Family intervention in psychosis 204
ALICIA STRINGFELLOW

Index *219*

List of editors and contributors

Nicola Evans is a senior lecturer in the School of Healthcare Sciences at Cardiff University.

Ben Hannigan is a reader in the School of Healthcare Sciences at Cardiff University.

Paul Bickerstaffe is a lecturer in the School of Healthcare Sciences at Cardiff University.

Elizabeth Bowring-Lossock is a lecturer in the School of Healthcare Sciences at Cardiff University.

Geoff Brennan is a mental health consultant and an executive director with Star Wards.

Sali Burns is a psychological therapist in Betsi Cadwaladr University Health Board.

Paul Cassedy is a lecturer in the School of Health Sciences at the University of Nottingham.

Billy Hardy is a senior lecturer in psychotherapy and a consultant systemic psychotherapist at the Family Institute in the University of South Wales.

Michelle Huws-Thomas is a lecturer in the School of Healthcare Sciences at Cardiff University.

John Hyde is a lecturer in the School of Healthcare Sciences at Cardiff University.

Gerwyn Jones is a lecturer in the School of Healthcare Sciences at Cardiff University.

Amanda King is a lecturer in the School of Healthcare Sciences at Cardiff University.

Jessica MacLaren is Post Doctoral Fellow in Nursing Studies in the School of Health in Social Science, University of Edinburgh.

Alex Nute is a lecturer in the School of Healthcare Sciences at Cardiff University.

Steven Pryjmachuk is Professor of Mental Health Nursing Education in the School of Nursing, Midwifery and Social Work at the University of Manchester.

Steve Riley is a consultant nurse in the North Wales Adolescent Mental Health Service in Betsi Cadwaladr University Health Board.

Iain Ryrie is a carer.

Theo Stickley is an associate professor in the School of Health Sciences at the University of Nottingham.

Alicia Stringfellow is a lecturer in the School of Healthcare Sciences at Cardiff University.

Jo Sullivan is a mental health nurse and cognitive behavioural therapist at the Forensic Service in Abertawe Bro Morgannwg University Health Board.

Norman Young is nurse consultant in Cardiff and Vale University Health Board and an associate lecturer in the School of Healthcare Sciences at Cardiff University.

Part 1
Foundations for practice

Preface

Introducing therapeutic skills

Nicola Evans and Ben Hannigan

In this preface we outline the hopes we have for our book, and how it might help mental health nurses engage in therapeutic work that people value. We also set out the book's structure. We think it important, however, to first say something about motivations for mental health nursing and to set the scene with some historical context.

Why do people become mental health nurses? In our experience it is the wish to help others recover from distress and ill-health, and to regain valued relationships with family, friends, colleagues and communities, that most attracts people to this field of work. Becoming, and remaining, a good mental health nurse takes time and effort, and demands a considered and reflective approach towards self and others. People making use of mental health nurses' time and expertise will often say it is the relationships they have with practitioners that are most appreciated. In modern systems of health and social care there is vital work to be done directed at the organisation, administration and coordination of services. This work often falls to nurses, but when tasks in these areas become too onerous, both nurses and the people they help feel keenly the loss of opportunity to spend therapeutic time together.

This idea that mental health nursing is about relationships with people has an honourable history. For example, in the early 1950s Hildegard Peplau wrote about the central place of interpersonal relations in nursing practice (Peplau, 1952, reprinted 1988). She emphasised the importance of skills, and founded a tradition of scholarship, practice and education concerned with the central, independent, therapeutic function of nurses. During the last half of the twentieth century the emergence of this therapeutic, interpersonal tradition within mental health nursing took place in a context of wider change. Important new ideas about people and society were appearing. Psychodynamic theories and practices showed how self-understanding and healing might be fostered through prolonged, interpersonal work with a skilled therapist. Behaviourists concerned themselves with observable human responses, and showed how people could be helped to learn new, healthier, ways of interacting. Humanistic thinkers suggested that each of us can grow and develop, the role of the skilled helper being to facilitate this through empathy and positive regard.

As Clarke (1999) has noted, foundational ideas of this type were influential across all of the helping professions, including mental health nursing. Peplau was informed by the work of US psychoanalyst Harry Stack Sullivan, but humanistic approaches were dominant by the time we (the two editors of this book) came to train for the profession. Curricula in the schools of nursing in which we, and countless others, learned were strongly influenced by the ideas of Carl Rogers. Over time, and certainly within the space of our careers, a remarkable variety of approaches to helping people have arisen and sometimes fused together. The evidence for this can be seen in the pages of this book. It has befitted mental health nursing to keep up to date with current thinking and new evidence of what is helpful to people in distress, and to incorporate the principles and practices into everyday work.

In recent years, we have observed (and thoroughly embrace) a move towards the promotion of recovery from mental illness. This implies new thinking on the part of nurses, and others working in the mental health field, towards an appreciation of the strengths and aspirations of people with lived experience of mental ill-health rather than their deficits and problems. In this text, we explore some therapeutic approaches that better equip mental health nurses to work collaboratively with people who access mental health services, to work together on enhancing strengths and promoting recovery.

With all this in mind, we hope that this edited text becomes the first – but never the last – book that students and novice practitioners of mental health nursing reach for to inform the development of their practical, face-to-face helping skills. We are also clear that this is not a book that will produce experts in any of the approaches described. We offer a series of theoretical and practical introductions, the skills outlined to be used with caution and always with expert supervision (see Chapter 2). For those seeking to become more advanced in specific aspects of their practice we commend suitably accredited, post-qualification education and training, and ongoing clinical supervision.

Our book is organised in three sections. Part 1 sets the foundations for practice, addressing essential areas of skill and knowledge for all mental health nurses, irrespective of their particular therapeutic orientation. This section includes this opening 'Introducing therapeutic skills' preface, a chapter on conducting assessment interviews, by Gerwyn Jones and Norman Young, and a chapter on clinical supervision, by Jessica MacClaren.

Part 2 focuses on therapeutic skills, covering a wide (but not exhaustive) range of approaches helpful with individuals experiencing a range of difficulties. Theo Stickley and Paul Cassedy open this section with a chapter on person-centred counselling, Nicola Evans addresses using a solution-focused approach and Michelle Huws-Thomas writes on motivational interviewing. Also in this section, Steven Pryjmachuk discusses using the skills of problem solving, John Hyde writes on the skill of offering psychoeducation and Joanne Sullivan on skills to challenge unhelpful thoughts. Paul Bickerstaffe and Amanda King contribute a chapter on validation skills applied to people with dementia, Iain Ryrie writes on preventing relapse and Geoff Brennan contributes on behavioural management/ activation. This, the longest section of the book, closes with Sali Burns and Steve Riley on mindfulness, and Elizabeth Bowring-Lossock on de-escalating volatile situations.

Part 3 extends to therapeutic approaches helpful with families and groups. Billy Hardy writes on working systemically with families in mind, Alex Nute on working with groups and Alicia Stringfellow closes the book with a chapter on family intervention in psychosis.

We very much hope that you enjoy, and learn from, this book. As editors we offer our thanks to the chapter contributors, and to Richard Townrow, Rachel Crookes and their colleagues at the Open University Press for their support for this project.

References

Clarke, L. (1999) *Challenging Ideas in Psychiatric Nursing.* London: Routledge.

Peplau, H. (1952, reprinted 1988) *Interpersonal Relations in Nursing.* Basingstoke: Macmillan.

1

Conducting assessment interviews

Gerwyn Jones and Norman Young

Introduction

An intrinsic component of mental health nursing practice is an initial assessment interview. This involves a discussion between the person using services and the nurse in a context of collaboration and mutual respect. It is through the initial assessment that the service user's initial needs can be identified. Through this process, the nurse is practising within the requirements of the Nursing and Midwifery Council (2010), which state that:

> All nurses in the UK at the point of registration [should be able] to work in partnership with individuals, carers and their families, to undertake a holistic, person centred and systematic assessment. This should incorporate physical, emotional, psychological, social, cultural, spiritual and risk related needs; which facilitates collaboration in the development of a comprehensive personalised plan of nursing care.
>
> (Essential skills cluster: Organisational aspects of care 12)

The aim of this chapter is to identify, describe and illustrate how to conduct mental health assessments in a collaborative way with people who access mental health services. The chapter will focus on the key learning objectives identified below, provide a step-by-step guide to conducting a holistic assessment, and draw on hypothetical material to demonstrate the skills required in this area, using specific clinical examples.

Learning objectives

After reading this chapter, you will be able to:

- describe the purpose of assessment

- describe an assessment framework for mental health nursing practice
- understand the knowledge and skills required to use the framework
- demonstrate how to use assessment skills.

What is meant by mental health assessment?

Assessment is the process of judging or estimating the value of something, articulated by Barker (2004) as: 'the decision-making process, based upon the collection of relevant information, using a formal set of ethical criteria, that contributes to an overall estimation of a person and his circumstances'.

The value of any quality such as a person's memory or their condition of housing, merits assessment in health settings because they enable the assessor to judge the person's state of health and the determinants of health. For instance, one way a person's health can be represented is by the absence of signs (visible to others) and symptoms (subjective experiences) of disease. Health and well-being has been described as feeling safe, satisfied and fulfilled (Stiglitz, Sen and Fitoussi, 2009; ONS, 2014). Therefore health can be influenced by social factors, 'determinants of health' that need to be considered when conducting a mental health assessment. These other factors, such as attitudes, social, economic and environmental factors (Marmot and Bell, 2012), may contribute to a person's experience of health, help seeking or approach to recovery. Mental health assessment is therefore concerned with the measurement of qualities that define what is mental health and well-being, alongside the variables that are important in cause, course and outcome. The scope of the assessment will be guided by the assessor's role, the context of their work, and the consumer preferences and responses of the service user.

Mental health assessment: the political, personal and interpersonal

The purpose and intended outcome of the assessment will ultimately guide what is assessed. Historically nursing assessments have focused on ascertaining the type and level of care and support that is required to enable the person to lead a fulfilling life. Since 1991, mental health nurses in England, Scotland and Wales have been guided in what to assess through the use of the Care Programme Approach (CPA) (Department of Health, 1990; Scottish Office, 1996; Welsh Assembly Government, 2003). Latterly, within Wales, CPA has been superseded by the introduction of care and treatment plans (CTPs) through the Mental Health (Wales) Measure (2010). In an effort to govern the work of clinicians, the bureaucracy of assessment and care planning has progressively grown over time. A further feature has been the inclusion of personalisation and the ethos of recovery in this process, reflecting the rising influence of service users in service design. Additionally, within England and Wales, the National Institute for Health and Care Excellence (NICE) provides clinical guidelines to support service users, carers and clinicians, in care and treatment planning for all the diagnostic categories of mental disorder, such as depression, anxiety, bipolar disorder and schizophrenia.

These instruments direct nurses to conduct comprehensive assessments, which include an assessment of mental health and aspects of an individual's functioning, including personal strengths, aspirations, supports and their environment. With this information nurses work with service users to co-produce a nursing care plan that usually sits within a multidisciplinary plan underpinned by a recovery ethos (Coombs, Crookes and Curtis, 2013).

When to conduct an assessment interview?

For this chapter we refer to the assessment interview as a formal meeting between a service user and a mental health nurse, in which a structured process of assessment takes place. Mental health nurses working across settings will be prompted to conduct an interview for the principal reasons that there has been a change in the person's presentation or circumstances, when the service user or their family request an assessment, or at a predetermined point in time, such as a follow-up or annual review. The context in which the mental health nurse and the service user meet will influence the number of opportunities for a formal interview as opposed to opportunistic assessments. Compare, for example, the three scenarios for the same service user presented in Box 1.1. In each situation it is timely to perform an assessment because of a change in presentation and scheduled reviews, but the person may not want or be able to engage in the process.

Box 1.1: Assessment opportunities

1. Kelvin is two days into his admission to an inpatient acute ward. He has been pacing around the ward, gesticulating to people and thin air, muttering to himself under his breath. Peter, his named nurse, invites Kelvin to sit down and talk, but Kelvin says that he does not want to and returns to his room.
2. Kelvin is five days into his admission. He has been pacing the ward and muttering to himself, but has been mixing with staff and other service users. Kelvin is invited to participate in a one-to-one session by his named nurse, Peter. Kelvin agrees and the two of them go to a consulting room where Peter is able to assess Kelvin's health and his needs, and they work on a collaborative plan of care.

3. Kelvin is ten days into his admission and is being supported by the home treatment team to spend overnight leave at his flat. Rachel and Tom from the home treatment team call on Kelvin for a scheduled appointment. Kelvin invites them in to his flat where they agree to assess his mental health, his living conditions and what he needs in order to enable him to be discharged from the hospital.

What to assess

The key features of a holistic mental health assessment are presented in Box 1.2. They are drawn from NICE guidance on service user experience, common mental disorders, and severe and enduring mental health problems (NICE, 2011a, 2011b, 2014). While the primary aim is to ascertain the person's care needs, nested within this is an assessment of risk. The National Patient Safety Agency identified that the risk areas that require assessment are those of suicide, self-harm, violence and aggression, dangerousness, self-neglect, physical and psychological abuse, and falls (NPSA, 2008).

Mental health nurses have a positive role in assessing common indicators of deteriorating physical health and acting as a facilitator for health promotion (Robson *et al.*, 2013). Such assessments are important because some mental health problems are associated with an increased risk of co-morbidities and early mortality (Cuijpers and Smit, 2002). For example, it is known that individuals diagnosed with schizophrenia and bipolar disorder die on average 15 years earlier than the general population (Crump, 2013).

Box 1.2: Areas of assessment

- Demographics: age, gender, ethnicity
- The person's personal perspective on, or narrative of, their experiences
- The presence of signs and symptoms of mental disorder (the mental state exam)
- History:
  - psychiatric history
  - physical history
  - personal history
  - family history
  - social history
  - forensic history
- Personality

- Risks:
  - suicide and self-harm
  - risk to others
  - risk from others (exploitation)
- Problems in functioning:
  - psychological functioning – intellectual, cognitive, emotional
  - social functioning – interpersonal, occupational
  - physical health
- Formal and informal needs and unmet needs
- Knowledge and understanding of their condition and needs
- Family and carers' knowledge and needs
- Strengths and abilities
- Goals and preferences

How to assess

Values and principles

Good assessments are achieved by adhering to the principles of the recovery approach (Repper and Perkins, 2003), where the development of collaborative partnership with the service user, their family or carer is combined with timely consultation with colleagues. Service users, their families and carers are often in a position of trying to cope with unusual and distressing circumstances in the best way they know how. Nurses need to be mindful of beliefs, attitudes and behaviours that may misinform the assessment and compromise trust. An example would be holding stereotypical attitudes or negative views towards service users diagnosed with personality disorders (Bodner, Cohen-Fridel and Iancu, 2011), leading to stigmatising and discriminatory practice (Thornicroft, 2006).

Preparation

Prior to starting an assessment you will need to identity what you will require to competently assess, and be prepared to document and communicate your findings to the service user and others. There may be specific templates that you need to use or you may be using assessment scales either on the day or given to the service user beforehand. You need to familiarise yourself with how to use standardised documentation and, in the case of specific measures, how to score, interpret and feed back the findings. Carpenter (2013, p. 53) identifies some tools that are of relevance for mental health nurses. These are summarised in Box 1.3.

Box: 1.3 Tools for assessment

Mood and anxiety

- Beck Depression Inventory II (BDI–II) (Beck *et al.*, 1996)
- Edinburgh Postnatal Depression Scale (EPDS) (Cox *et al.*, 1987)
- Generalised Anxiety Disorder Assessment (GAD-7) (Spitzer *et al.*, 2006)
- Geriatric Depression Scale (short form) (GDS) (Hoyle *et al.*, 1999)
- Patient Health Questionnaire (PHQ-9) (Kroenke *et al.*, 2001)
- Hamilton Anxiety Scale (HAS) (Hamilton, 1969)

General assessment

- Brief Psychiatric Rating Scale (BPRS) (Lukoff *et al.*, 1986)
- General Health Questionnaire (GHQ) (Goldberg and Williams, 1988)
- Instrumental and Expressive Functions of Social Support (IEFSS) (Ensel and Woelfel, 1986)

Psychosis

- Positive and Negative Symptom Scale (PANSS) (Kay *et al.*, 1988)

Allocating time to prepare for new service users or service users undergoing a review is an important consideration. Gathering relevant historical information on the person's mental health, functioning and risk will allow you to target your line of questions, choose appropriate measures, avoid repetition, anticipate sensitive areas of enquiry, and enable you to demonstrate understanding and interest in the person. It is equally important to consider whether it is pertinent to commence a clinical assessment by considering a service user's previous history or to start with the current precipitating factors. However, one needs to be mindful that attending to previous history is not just about reading a service user's notes (Carpenter, 2013). The key is to contextualise current issues through the establishment of a timeline of events that led to the current presentation – this will include issues of risk to the individual or others.

Structuring

Mental health assessments can be structured as in initial assessments or reviews, or they can be informal, observational and opportunistic, such as the daily assessment on an inpatient ward. In more formal circumstances, such as an interview, service users can often be concerned about what will happen, how long it will take and what will happen afterwards. Being able to convey to the person the purpose, nature and duration of the meeting is advantageous as it allows for a collaborative and informed meeting to take place. The context in which the assessment happens is important in creating an environment where privacy is maintained and where individuals are happy to divulge personal information.

An overview of the interview structure is given in Box 1.4 and is drawn from good practice in consulting with service users (Hastings and Redsell, 2006; NICE, 2011b).

Box 1.4: Interview structure

1. Relationship building
    a. Introductions and pleasantries
    b. Agenda setting: agreeing the content, progression and the timings of the assessment
    c. Defining the boundaries of the meeting, including confidentiality and information sharing
2. Gathering information
    a. Use open and closed questions to fulfil the purpose of the interview
    b. Administer measures or scales
    c. Provide information and answer the service user's questions
3. Formulation
    a. Prioritising areas of concern or areas of focus
    b. Shared decision making and action planning
4. Closing
    a. Giving and eliciting feedback
    b. Deciding on follow-up
5. Sharing information with other people

Relationship building

As with any nursing interaction, when first meeting a service user it is important to introduce yourself and state your role. Most importantly, nurses need to be able to actively engage with a service user to develop an equal and trusting relationship that promotes hope and optimism (Hastings and Redsell, 2006). Relationship building encompasses the concept of engagement, which involves the skills of demonstrating empathy, attending to the service user, and having a respectful and compassionate attitude (Roberts, 2013). As with any professional interaction we must outline how information will be shared, and be mindful of professional boundaries as set out by the Nursing and Midwifery Council (2015).

All nursing work is sensitive to time constraints, and interviewing is no different. New referrals from primary health care can demand up to an hour and a half including documentation, while a routine follow-up and review at a person's home may take 50 minutes. Irrespective of the context, the interviewer is concerned with the length of time required to collect the right amount of information (sufficiency) in the shortest amount of time (efficiency).

Agreeing how long you have together and how the meeting will progress is a useful technique to allow the pace of the session to be set. The example in Box 1.5 is divided into two sections. First, the nurse sets out the purpose of the meeting and implicitly leads the conversation, but offers the service user an opportunity during the conversation to gain feedback and clarify understanding. The nurse proceeds to provide information about how they would like the interview to progress before handing back to the service user to enable them to co-produce the agenda.

Box 1.5: Setting a collaborative agenda for an interview

Nurse: Mr Patel, I am Jane, a mental health nurse. I am pleased that you have been able to come to the community centre today and trust that you found the directions helpful?

Mr Patel: Yes it was easy to find.

Nurse: Good. I understand the main reason for meeting with me today is to assess concerns you have that may relate to your mental health.

Mr Patel: Yes, I saw my GP and she said I should see you … I can't sleep properly, can't get these images out of my mind.

Nurse: You have some problems with sleeping and images; before we look at them in detail I'd just like to outline how I'd like to go about the assessment and make sure I cover everything that is important for you. I want to use 60 minutes to ask some questions about your main problems, and then move on to ask some things about you and any past treatment you may have had, before moving on to check how you have been feeling over the last week. Finally, and if appropriate for you, I'd like to talk about what the best kind of help would be. What we talk about will be in confidence and at the end I'd like to make sure you are happy on what to share with your GP or anyone else. Would that be OK?

Mr Patel: That sounds fine.

Nurse: Is there anything else that you think it is important we cover?

Mr Patel: No, all that is fine.

Gathering information

In interviews questions can be used to explore the qualities of a subjective experience, such as a type of thinking and emotions or objective phenomenon such as behaviour. Acquiring a balance of objective and subjective data by capturing an individual's experience (Greenhalgh, 2006) aids this process and ensures that the assessment is not merely an unsophisticated exchange of information (Roberts, 2013).

Across the areas of assessment described in Box 1.2 the interviewer will need to use open questions to draw out relevant information. Open questions are usually prefaced by who, what, when, why, where or how. These are the '5Ws' demonstrated in Box 1.6. Here the interviewer is interested in determining what level of need the person has in using transport. Note that, towards the conclusion of the conversation, the interviewer uses a hypothetical situation to explore what the person would do if the problem of using transport was resolved or if they were given help. This allows the interviewer to demonstrate understanding and aid clarification through the use of reflection and summaries. This is illustrated at the end of the dialogue in Box 1.6, when the interviewer is considering moving on to the next topic.

Box 1.6 The 5Ws

Open questions

Nurse: What help do you need, if any, in using public transport?

Service user: I rarely use the bus or train at all.

Nurse: Why is that?

Service user: I get confused about the times and don't like the crowds – it feels like they are staring at me.

Nurse: How do you travel from place to place now?

Service user: I occasionally use taxis but mainly get lifts from my family if I need to do any shopping. Using taxis gets expensive and I don't like to keep asking my family.

Nurse: Who do you rely on?

Service user: My sister mainly, she works part-time and gives me a lift once a week to go to the supermarket.

Nurse: Just imagining that you were able to use public transport, where would you go?

Service user: I could go to the clothes shops, not just the supermarket, or visit the cinema.

Nurse: So at the moment you get help from your sister to shop once a week, otherwise you will use taxis, but you tend to avoid this because it is expensive. You find it difficult to use public transport because you find it confusing and you get anxious fearing people are staring at you. If you were able to use public transport you could go to the cinema or clothes shopping.

When undertaking an assessment we not only need to identify what the individual is experiencing (e.g. hearing voices) but also to quantify this experience in some way. Again questions can be utilised to elicit the frequency, the intensity (or strength), preoccupation (how difficult it is to move one's attention away from the experience) the duration (how long before it goes away) and occurrence (when it is more likely to occur). In Box 1.7 the nurse is interested in working with the service user on their voice hearing, and wishes to quantify the experience so that any interventions can be evaluated in the future. Note that the nurse is not assessing the content of the voice hearing or the impact of the experience on the voice hearer.

Box 1.7: Using questions to quantify

Nurse: James, how often do you hear the voice?
Service user: Through the week really, most days.
Nurse: Would you say more often than not in the week?
Service user: Yes, most days.
Nurse: And on those days how often through the day?
Service user: Maybe once, maybe twice, but no more than that.
Nurse: When the voice speaks, how loud is it? For example, a whisper, general speech, loud speech or shouting.
Service user: Sort of normal speech but it is distracting.
Nurse: How difficult is it to move your attention away from the voice?
Service user: Not too hard. It is distracting to begin with, but when I concentrate on other things it goes into the background.
Nurse: When you're not distracted how long is it before the voice goes away?
Service user: About 15 to 20 minutes.
Nurse: Have you noticed when you are more likely to hear the voice?
Service user: Usually at night time.

Formulation

Following the assessment the nurse and service user interpret the data and prioritise areas of concern or areas of focus in the shape of a formulation. Look at the scenario in Box 1.8.

Box 1.8: Formulation

John is 22 years old and lives at home with his parents. He works at a local supermarket and has a steady girlfriend. John has a diagnosis of clinical depression and is under the care of his local general practitioner (GP). Recently his mood has deteriorated considerably and John has been referred by his GP to the Primary Mental Health Team for assessment. John is reported to be very low in mood, and states that he has no enjoyment in life. His sleep has become increasingly disturbed, while his appetite has diminished and he experiences fatigue and poor concentration. As a result John is off sick from work and has become more isolated at home.

The questioning approaches described above can be used to help John develop a statement that describes the impact of the experience of depression on his lifestyle. This should be written in his words to reduce the use of jargon and to provide individual meaning for John, as well as identifying observable behaviours (see Box 1.9).

Box 1.9: Describing the impact of experiences

Nurse: John, in terms of your mental health, how would you describe your main problem at the moment?

John: My main problem is my low mood, which has come on over the past three months. I've got no energy, get tired out really easily, I've lost my appetite and can't sleep. I find myself crying for no reason, and sometimes I just spend the day in bed. I am off sick as I just can't face the stress of work. I've stopped seeing friends, lost interest in going to the gym, and me and my girlfriend are not getting on at the moment.

The nurse and John are now in a position to reframe this statement as a series of needs. These can subsequently be translated into SMART (specific, measurable, achievable, realistic, time-bound) goals in the form of an action plan. This process ensures that decision making is shared and allows John to prioritise the goals he wants to work towards, as shown in Box 1.10.

Box: 1.10: SMART goals and action plans

Nurse: So, John, if I can just summarise my understanding of what we have discussed. Your main problem is your low mood, which has come on over the past three months. You have no energy, you get tired easily, you have lost your appetite and can't sleep. You often cry for no reason and spend the day in bed. You are off sick as you can't face the stress of work and you have stopped seeing your friends. You have lost interest in your hobbies and you are not getting on at the moment with your girlfriend.

John: Yes I think that sums it up.

Nurse: So what would need to change for these issues to no longer be a problem?

John: I need to sleep properly – that would make me less tired and agitated.

Nurse: Is there anything else that needs to change?

John: I need to be able to exercise, which will also improve my mood and make me feel more motivated.

Nurse: John we have established that you want to return to a regular sleep pattern, which before your depression involved you getting about seven hours' sleep a night. If we are to set a goal to meet your need how can we phrase this?

John: I would like to improve my sleep pattern so I am consistently achieving seven hours per night.

Nurse: What about exercising? Previously you attended the gym about four days a week. What do you think is reasonable to start you back?

John: I would like to start exercising twice a week.

Closing

On completion of the assessment the nurse should begin to close the meeting by providing feedback that is tailored to the service user through consideration of their preferences, their capacity to comprehend complex versus simple information, and their strengths and abilities. Such information will include:

- how the nurse understands the problem
- what the nurse considers are the next best steps
- integration of the service user's expectations, values and strengths
- how the information will be shared.

With the assessment and planning over it is often helpful to elicit feedback from the service user about their experience of the interview. The purpose of this is to develop insights into any material that was missed and to look for any opportunities to improve practice. Two simple questions may suffice:

1. Was there anything helpful about meeting today?
2. Was there anything that was unhelpful?

Finally, the nurse may need to identify a follow-up date, and the assessment should be recorded in relevant documentation and shared. In deciding when to reassess, a useful question will be 'How long will it be before a change will occur?' Where the person's mental state may fluctuate rapidly, then it may be reasonable to review them the next day. In a community setting, a change may not be expected for two weeks.

Sharing information

While consent to obtain information will have been gained at the outset of the interview, gaining consent on how it will be shared is necessary at the end.

The assessor will need to communicate the content and outcome decisions of the assessment to other relevant clinicians and family or carers. Such communication may involve handover to colleagues in an inpatient setting, feeding back to the service user's GP by letter following an assessment, or to other teams or agencies by phone. A discussion of what can be conveyed, i.e. general or specific information, and to whom, i.e. professional and or relatives and carers, will allow the service user to be in control of the use of their information (NICE, 2011b). Sometimes gaining consent will not be possible – for example, when the person lacks mental capacity or they present a danger to themselves and others but do not want their information shared. At these times local policies and procedures, as well as professional guidance on confidentiality, should be consulted (Nursing and Midwifery Council, 2015).

Families and carers will also want to know the outcome of the assessment and, in situations where service users are reluctant to share information, it is worth asking whether general rather than specific details can be shared (Worthington, Rooney and Hannan, 2013). For example, the service user may consent to sharing that 'he is anxious and angry because he feels that people are getting at him at the moment', in preference to 'he is anxious and angry at you because he thinks that you may be poisoning his food'.

A useful tool for communicating verbal information is SBAR (Box 1.11), an easy-to-remember mechanism for framing communications (Velji *et al.*, 2008).

Box 1.11: SBAR: Situation–Background–Assessment–Recommendation

S – Situation: what is happening at the present time?

B – Background: what are the circumstances leading up to this situation?

A – Assessment: what do I think the problem is?

R – Recommendation: what should we do to correct the problem?

Conclusion

Interviewing skills are usually called upon during the assessment phases in mental health care. The purpose of assessment is to judge the quality or value of something. For mental health nurses this is commonly a person's mental health, well-being and needs. Depending on the context of the assessment and the role of the nurse, the interview can extend into assessing the determinants of health, such as a detailed assessment of the person's social circumstances. Assessment interviews follow the process of relationship building, gathering information, formulating, closing, and sharing information. In demonstrating competence in interviewing, nurses draw on skills in relationship building, questioning, formulating, and demonstrating understanding by providing feedback, and collaboration through shared decision making and sharing information. The outcome of a good interview will allow care planning to progress in a timely and effective manner for the benefit of the service user, their family or carers and other team members.

Activities

Activity 1: audio recording
If possible obtain the permission of a service user to record your next assessment. When reviewing the interview, analyse how you move from section to section of the assessment, how you used questions to elicit information and how you provided feedback about the assessment findings.

Activity 2: peer review
Ask a mentor or more experienced nurse to sit in on your assessment and provide feedback on your knowledge and skills.

Activity 3: not using certain phrases
Become aware of phrases you may overuse by deliberately stopping using them. For example, to avoid leading questions, write on a piece of paper the phrase 'do you' to remind yourself not to use sentences that start with the phrase. Try others, such as 'were you', or ones you may tend to repeat – for example, 'How did you feel?'

Suggested reading

Norman, I.J. and Ryrie, I. (2013) Assessment, in Norman, I. and Ryrie I. (eds) *The Art and Science of Mental Health Nursing*, 3rd edn. Maidenhead: Open University Press.

This is a good, easy-to-read overview of the rationale for assessment, and incudes further discussion of useful measures.

References

Barker, P.J. (2004) *Assessment in Psychiatric and Mental Health Nursing: In Search of the Whole Person*, 2nd edn. Cheltenham: Nelson Thornes.
Bodner, E., Cohen-Fridel, S. and Iancu, I. (2011) Staff attitudes toward patients with borderline personality disorder. *Comprehensive Psychiatry*, 52, 548–555.
Carpenter, D. (2013) Types of assessment, in Walker, S., Carpenter, D. and Middlewick, Y. (eds) *Assessment and Decision Making in Mental Health Nursing* (pp. 39–55). London: Sage.
Coombs, T., Crookes, P. and Curtis, J. (2013) A comprehensive mental health nursing assessment: variability of content in practice: content assessment. *Journal of Psychiatric and Mental Health Nursing*, 20, 150–155.

Crump, C. (2013) Comorbidities and mortality in persons with schizophrenia: a Swedish national cohort study. *American Journal of Psychiatry*, 170, 3, 324–333.

Cuijpers, P. and Smit, F. (2002) Excess mortality in depression: a meta-analysis of community studies. *Journal of Affective Disorders*, 72, 227–236.

Department of Health (1990) Care Programme Approach Circular HC(90)23/LASSL(90)11. London: Department of Health.

Greenhalgh, T. (2006) *What Seems to be the Trouble? Stories in Illness and Healthcare.* Oxford: Radcliffe Publishing Ltd.

Hastings, A. and Redsell, S. (2006) *The Good Consultation Guide for Nurses.* Abingdon: Radcliffe Publishing Ltd.

Marmot, M. and Bell, R. (2012) Fair society, healthy lives. *Public Health*, 126, September, Suppl. 1: S4–10.

Mental Health (Wales) (2010) *Measure 2010.* Neath Port Talbot: Mental Health (Wales).

NICE (2011a) *Common Mental Health Disorders* (CG123). London: National Institute for Health and Clinical Excellence.

NICE (2011b) *Service User Experience in Adult Mental Health* (CG136). London: National Institute for Health and Clinical Excellence.

NICE (2014) *Psychosis and Schizophrenia in Adults: Treatment and Management* (CG178). London: National Institute for Health and Care Excellence.

NPSA (2008) *Seven Steps to Patient Safety in Mental Health.* London: National Patient Safety Agency.

Nursing and Midwifery Council (2015) *The Code: Professional standards of practice and behaviour for nurses and midwives.* London: Nursing and Midwifery Council.

ONS (2014) National well-being measures, March. London: Office for National Statistics.

Repper, J. and Perkins, R. (2003) *Social Inclusion and Recovery: A Model for Mental Health Practice.* Edinburgh and New York: Baillière Tindall.

Roberts, D. (2013) *Psychosocial Nursing Care a Guide to Nursing the Whole Person.* Berkshire: Open University Press.

Robson, D., Haddad, M., Gray, R. and Gournay, K. (2013) Mental health nursing and physical health care: a cross-sectional study of nurses' attitudes, practice, and perceived training needs for the physical health care of people with severe mental illness. *International Journal of Mental Health Nursing*, 22, 409–417.

Scottish Office (1996) Community care: care programme approach for people with severe and enduring mental illness including dementia. Circular no. SWSG16/96.

Stiglitz, J.E., Sen, A. and Fitoussi, J.-P. (2009) *Report of the Commission on the Measurement of Economic Performance and Social Progress.* Paris: Commission on the Measurement of Economic Performance and Social Progress.

Thornicroft, G. (2006) *Shunned: Discrimination Against People with Mental Illness.* Oxford and New York: Oxford University Press.

Velji, K., Baker, G.R., Fancott, C., Andreoli, A., Boaro, N., Tardif, G., Aimone, E. and Sinclair, L. (2008) Effectiveness of an adapted SBAR communication tool for a rehabilitation setting. *Healthcare Quarterly*, 11, 72–79.

Welsh Assembly Government (2003) *Mental Health Policy Wales: Implementation Guidance – The Care Programme Approach for Mental Health Service Users.* Cardiff: Welsh Assembly Government.

Worthington, A., Rooney, P. and Hannan, R. (2013) *The Triangle of Care*, 2nd edn. London: Carers Trust.

2

Clinical supervision

Jessica MacLaren

Introduction

This chapter explores *supervision,* a flexible practice, which is used to develop and maintain the interpersonal, therapeutic and professional skills of mental health nurses. The chapter begins by discussing what is meant by the term supervision, and how it is used in mental health nursing. It then goes on to explore the supervision relationship and some of the key elements of supervision, before addressing issues to consider when establishing supervision practice.

Learning objectives

After reading this chapter, you will:

- understand how and why supervision is used in mental health nursing
- understand the roles of supervisee and supervisor
- identify key elements of supervision, and different approaches to these
- recognise issues to be considered when engaging in supervision.

Supervision in mental health nursing

Supervision in mental health care has been around for more than a century, and disciplines such as counselling, psychoanalysis, clinical psychology and social work have developed distinctive, yet cross-fertilising, traditions of supervision (Carroll, 2007; Bernard and Goodyear, 2014). In mental health nursing, supervision developed relatively recently, and has been influenced by practices in other disciplines (Butterworth, 1992; Sloan, 2006). There is consequently no single model of supervision in mental health nursing, and instead mental health nurses may use a variety of approaches that come under the heading 'supervision'.

Understandably, this variety of approaches can lead to confusion about what is actually meant by supervision, and it is perhaps most helpful to begin by thinking of supervision as an umbrella term, covering different but overlapping practices, which generally involve:

> a semi-structured process where a mental health nurse (the supervisee) meets regularly and confidentially with a more experienced practitioner (the supervisor) to discuss issues of relevance to the supervisee's practice.
>
> (Cleary, Horsfall and Happell, 2010, p. 525)

Why do supervision?

Kalpna is a student nurse on placement in a psychiatric admissions ward. She is asked to look after a young woman, Bridget, who is withdrawn and depressed. Kalpna gets on well with Bridget, who opens up to her about some distressing childhood experiences. After their conversation Bridget thanks Kalpna for her support, and Kalpna feels satisfied that they have established a good relationship. Later that day, however, Kalpna learns that Bridget has cut herself badly. She is shocked and distressed. She doesn't understand why Bridget didn't ask her for help, and worries that their conversation may have caused Bridget to self-harm.

Mental health nurses work with individuals who suffer from psychological and emotional disorders, and as in Kalpna's story, this kind of work can evoke confusing and distressing emotions that are difficult to process in day-to-day practice. Mental health nurses also work on a complex interpersonal level, requiring a high level of critical self-awareness in order to engage therapeutically with each unique service user. Supervision can be a foundation that supports this complex work, facilitating the development and practice of interpersonal and therapeutic skills, as Hawkins and Shohet (2012, p. 60) describe here:

> Supervision is a joint endeavour in which a practitioner with the help of a supervisor, attends to their service users, themselves as part of their client practitioner relationships and the wider systemic context, and by so doing improves the quality of their work, transforms their client relationships, continuously develops themselves, their practice and the wider profession.

Supervision is commonly regarded as performing a mixture of educational, quality control, developmental and supportive functions, and one or other of these functions may be given greater emphasis at any given time or in a particular form of supervision (Proctor, 2001; Bernard and Goodyear, 2014).

There are a growing number of studies that seek to evaluate the effectiveness of supervision in performing various functions, and there is evidence that supervision has a positive effect on nurses' well-being, and may contribute to the quality of nursing practice (for example, see Hyrkäs, Appelqvist-Schmidlechner and Oksa, 2003; Hyrkäs, 2005; Edwards *et al.*, 2006; Bradshaw, Butterworth and Mairs, 2007; Koivu, Saarinen and Hyrkas, 2012). Overall, however, much of the thinking around how and why mental nurses should do supervision is theoretical, and there is evidence that in practice supervision often falls short of the ideal (cf. Sloan, 2006; White and Winstanley, 2010). Perhaps the most convincing arguments for supervision come from scholars and practitioners who write from their own extensive experience of participating in supervision:

> supervision interrupts practice. It wakes us up to what we are doing, we wake up to what it is, instead of falling asleep in the comfort stories of our clinical routines.
>
> (Ryan 2004, cited in Carroll, 2007, p. 36)

Activity 1 in Box 2.1 invites you to return to Kalpna and Bridget, and to consider the effects of the different approaches which Kalpna's supervisor could take.

Box 2.1 Activity 1

Think about what functions supervision might perform when Kalpna discusses Bridget with her supervisor, George. How do you think each of the three approaches described below might help Kalpna? Which do you think is the most useful? Are there any other approaches George could take?

1. George encourages Kalpna to think about how she could have better assessed Bridget's level of risk. Had she read Bridget's notes and care plans before talking to her, and did she ask Bridget if she felt like self-harming?
2. George explains to Kalpna that Bridget's self-harming is a coping strategy, and suggests some books she could read about self-harm. They agree that future supervision sessions will focus on Kalpna's work with service users who self-harm, and she will keep a diary of her work with these service users, and bring this to supervision.
3. George encourages Kalpna to express how she feels about Bridget's behaviour. Kalpna tells George that she feels guilty, and blames herself for causing Bridget to self-harm. At the same time she feels angry and hurt by Bridget, who she feels rejected her attempts to help. George and Kalpna discuss how these feelings are affecting her relationship with Bridget and with other service users. They also talk about Kalpna's expectations of herself as a nurse, and how these influence the way she responded to the situation.

The supervision relationship

At the heart of supervision is the relationship between *supervisor* (the person who listens and responds to the supervisee) and *supervisee* (the person whose work is discussed in supervision), and it is arguably this relationship that makes supervision unique. This section explores these two roles, and how they may be enacted in different ways.

The supervisor's role

A supervisor may or may not be a mental health nurse. Often the supervisor is selected on the basis that they are an *expert*. They may have expertise in a particular clinical area, or they may be an expert *in supervision*, being skilled at facilitating the interpersonal and reflective process of supervision (Jones, 1998).

Sometimes the supervisor is in a position of power, as a senior practitioner who evaluates the supervisee's work and teaches best practice (Bernard and Goodyear, 2014). Alternatively, the supervisor may work in partnership with the supervisee, who is positioned as the expert on their own practice while the supervisor facilitates a relational reflective process (Frawley-O'Dea and Sarnat, 2001). In nursing, the role of supervisor is sometimes performed by the nurse's line manager; this is widely criticised as creating a hierarchical relationship that inhibits a reflective, supportive discussion, and moves the focus of supervision onto managerial concerns (Yegdich, 1999; Sloan, 2006).

The role of the supervisor is key in determining what is discussed in supervision. For example, in each of the scenarios above, George takes a different approach to Kalpna's problem, focusing variously on practical clinical skills, education and interpersonal processes. The approach taken by the supervisor is likely to be influenced by his/her own professional background and interests. Some supervisors may focus on teaching knowledge and skills to their supervisee, others may be more interested in discussing diagnosis and treatment, while some may focus on the thoughts, feelings and experiences of the supervisee her/himself (Frawley-O'Dea and Sarnat, 2001).

Being a supervisee

The supervisor's approach and actions strongly influence the course of supervision, but the role of supervisee is equally important in establishing a good relationship and constructing productive supervision practice. As Rodgers and Shohet describe here, being a supervisee can be rewarding:

> To be a supervisee has meant being in a place of support, challenge and growth. My first supervisor had to somewhat straddle the roles of therapist and supervisor. I remember clearly I needed to be taken under somebody's wing. As a supervisee I revel in space provided for me. I care deeply about

my work, my clients, and it's wonderful to have a place to share this love of being human, with all its struggles.

(Rodgers and Shohet, 2011, p. 109)

The relational nature of supervision means that it is important that the novice supervisee chooses a supervisor who has the requisite skills and experience to ensure that their supervision practice is safe and productive. At the same time it is also important for the supervisee to take an active part in constructing their supervision practice, ensuring that it meets their needs and does not cross personal boundaries. As Rodgers and Shohet observe, above, it can sometimes be difficult to separate supervision from therapy, given that in many forms of supervision the supervisee discusses how their own thoughts, emotions and history influence their response to a service user (Frawley-O'Dea and Sarnat, 2001; Bernard and Goodyear, 2014).

Activity 2 in Box 2.2 introduces you to Colin and Laura, and asks you to reflect on the boundaries between personal experiences and professional practice.

Box 2.2 Activity 2

Think about the questions below in relation to the following scenario:

As Colin discusses a case with his supervisor, Laura, it becomes clear that this service user's marital difficulties remind Colin of his own painful divorce some years ago, and this is having an effect on Colin's approach to his service user. Laura reflects this back to Colin, asking about the feelings he is still dealing with in the wake of his divorce. Colin replies that he realises his feelings are influencing the nurse–service user relationship, but they are too difficult for him to talk about in supervision.

1. What might be the advantages and disadvantages of Colin talking about his feelings around marriage and divorce?
2. How could Laura and Colin work in a way that is supportive and productive?
3. To what extent would you be willing to talk about personal feelings and history in supervision?
4. What boundaries would you wish to establish in your supervision?

Key elements of supervision

This section considers some of the key elements of supervision. Different approaches to supervision may give greater emphasis to one or more of these elements.

Time

One of the most important characteristics of supervision is continuity over time. Supervision relationships can be open ended, and nurses may engage in supervision

throughout their careers. The continuing nature of supervision allows for the creation of a trusting, evolving relationship between supervisor and supervisee (Bernard
and Goodyear, 2014), but it also means that supervision needs are likely to change
over time. This may mean looking for a supervisor with expertise in a particular
area or, alternatively, some experienced practitioners prefer a more egalitarian form
of supervision in which supervisee and supervisor are peers (cf. Stevenson and
Jackson, 2000). The long-term nature of supervision means that it is important for
supervisor and supervisee to regularly review and discuss changing needs.

Reflection

Reflection-on-action – 'the ability to think about the past, in the present for the
future' (Carroll, 2011, p. 19) – is widely regarded as the mechanism of supervision.
Reflection uncovers knowledge that practitioners may not be consciously aware
they possess, facilitating experiential learning and fostering critical self-awareness
(Schön, 1983). In supervision, the supervisee reflects on, and learns from, their past
experience of practice, and uses this learning to inform future practice.

As with supervision, there are many different models and approaches to
reflection, but the process begins with the practitioner recounting an experience (Schön, 1983; Rolfe, Freshwater and Jasper, 2001). A supervisor may then
encourage their supervisee to think more deeply, perhaps by asking questions
about the reasons for certain actions, thoughts or feelings, or by connecting the
specific experience to a wider context or history (Rolfe *et al.*, 2001). This can be
a challenging process, disrupting established ways of thinking, and so it is important to ensure reflection in supervision is both emotionally safe and productive
(Todd and Freshwater, 1999; Johns, 2006).

Activity 3 in Box 2.3 invites you to practise reflection-on-action and to consider what you have learned as a result.

Box 2.3 Activity 3

Practise reflecting-on-action
- Ensure you have time and privacy for this exercise.
- Choose an experience on which you would like to reflect.
- Write down the story of this experience, being as detailed as possible.
- Read over what you have written.
- Ask yourself questions (e.g. what was most important/uncomfortable/mem-
  orable about the experience? Have your feelings changed over time? Does
  the experience compare to past events? Did it change your future actions?).
- Use your imagination to think about the experience in different ways, e.g. by
  writing an account from the perspective of one of the other people there, or
  different ways the events could have happened.
- Finally, think about the reflective process in which you have just engaged.
  How did it feel? Did you learn anything? What did you like/dislike about it?

Learning

Learning is a major aim of supervision, and typically takes place through the process of reflection (although learning in supervision can also follow a tutorial or training format) (Hawkins and Shohet, 2012; Bernard and Goodyear, 2014). Learning can occur on different levels, from basic problem solving, to deeply self-reflective learning that engages with difficult emotions like uncertainty and shame (Carroll, 2011).

Emotions

Emotions enter supervision in different ways. They enter through practice; mental health nurses work with the emotions of others on a daily basis, and the therapeutic use of self requires nurses to work with their own emotions (Freshwater, 2002; Norman and Ryrie, 2013). They also enter through the empathic connection between supervisee and supervisor (Hawkins and Shohet, 2012), and through the emotional process of reflective learning (Carroll, 2011; Bernard and Goodyear, 2014).

Supervision may involve the discussion and expression of uncomfortable emotions (e.g. when Kalpna admits to feeling angry with Bridget). Emotionally safe and skilfully facilitated supervision can help nurses to enter into a more open and progressive dialogue with difficult feelings and experiences, allowing them to process and learn from these experiences (Ryde, 2011).

Monitoring

Sometimes the supervisor is expected to monitor the supervisee's quality or safety of practice, and even where the supervisor has no direct monitoring function they always have a duty to respond to situations where the supervisee or their service user may be at risk (Hawkins and Shohet, 2012). Furthermore, the very nature of supervision opens the supervisee's practice up to scrutiny, which can be both ethically desirable and emotionally exposing (Gilbert, 2001; Clouder and Sellars, 2004; Buus *et al.*, 2011).

Supervision below the surface

In relationships there can be processes happening of which we are not overtly aware, and we may pick up on emotional echoes from other people (Frosh, 2012). For example, imagine you and I are talking casually about something when you suddenly start to feel sad for no apparent reason. Puzzled, you wonder why you feel sad, what has caused the sadness? When a seemingly inexplicable emotion appears like this during an interaction you may be picking up on something that *I* am feeling. Perhaps I am feeling sad, and although I do not overtly express this sadness, it is communicated to you *below the surface* of our conversation. Neither of us is consciously aware of what is happening, but you can feel the echo of my emotion in your body.

In interpersonal work it can be helpful to develop an understanding of these kinds of below-the-surface processes. Reflecting on the therapeutic relationship can build awareness of these processes, allowing you to develop a deeper understanding about what is going on between you and your service user (Frawley-O'Dea and Sarnat, 2001).

> *Ron is meeting a new service user, Linda, for the first time. Within moments of their meeting, Ron experiences a strong feeling of dislike towards Linda. He is troubled by this as it is unusual for him to have such a negative reaction to a service user and the dislike he feels makes it difficult for him to establish a good relationship with Linda.*
>
> *Ron discusses the case with his supervisor, who suggests that he may be experiencing an echo of Linda's own feelings about herself. Linda believes that other people dislike her, and this has been re-created in her relationship with Ron. Once Ron becomes aware of this process he is able to work through his feelings of dislike, and bring awareness of this to his work with Linda.*

Supervision can be thought of as involving two relationships (*Service user+Nurse* and *Nurse+Supervisor*), and relationally oriented approaches to supervision view these relationships as operating in parallel (Frawley-O'Dea and Sarnat, 2001). Thus processes that occur in the *Service user+Nurse* relationship may be re-enacted in the *Nurse+Supervisor* relationship. If the nurse and supervisor are willing to reflect openly and honestly about how *they* experience *their* relationship, then they may uncover important clues about the service user's feelings.

In the scenario above, Ron finds his dislike for Linda inexplicable, and discusses it openly with his supervisor. However, in a slightly different scenario, Ron may be unable to bring himself to consciously acknowledge his difficult feelings towards Linda, and instead they are suppressed. When he subsequently discusses Linda's case with his supervisor he does not identify these suppressed feelings, instead communicating them to his supervisor below the surface. Suddenly his supervisor has an inexplicable feeling of intense dislike towards Ron! A self-aware supervisor will reflect on this feeling, question its origin, and reflect on it with Ron: 'When you talk about Linda, I'm aware of strongly negative feelings, does that resonate with you?' In this way Ron and his supervisor become aware of an interpersonal process that might otherwise have continued unexplored, and may have sabotaged Ron's therapeutic relationship with Linda.

The kind of process occurring here between Linda, Ron and his supervisor is called a *parallel process*, describing the way in which what happens in the supervision relationship can sometimes mimic the therapeutic relationship. This term is used in counselling and psychotherapy supervision, but has also been adopted in nursing supervision (Playle and Mullarkey, 1998). Counsellors and psycho-therapists may also think about below-the-surface processes using concepts such as *countertransference, empathy* or *projective identification* to describe what is happening between therapist and service user (Frosh, 2012; McLeod, 2013).

In order to work with below-the-surface processes in supervision, the super-visor must be familiar with working in this way as it requires a high level of self-awareness, and can be a challenging experience, particularly if the supervisee has never engaged in personal therapy (Frawley-O'Dea and Sarnat, 2001). It is therefore essential for the supervisee to attend to the thoughts and feelings that supervision evokes.

Practicalities

Engaging in supervision involves addressing practical considerations such as how often, for how long and where supervision is carried out (cf. Hyrkäs, 2005; Edwards *et al.*, 2006). Choosing one's own supervisor, managerial support for supervision, consistency and continuity, and having adequate time and space, all impact on the quality of supervision (cf. Cleary and Freeman, 2005, Hyrkäs, 2005). Nurses attempting to establish a supervision practice may encounter obstacles such as a lack of experienced and qualified supervisors, and the dif-ficulty of keeping protected time for supervision.

When preparing for supervision it will be helpful to research relevant con-cepts and practices. There is a large body of literature on supervision (see the 'Suggested reading' and 'References' at the end of this chapter for suggestions), and some universities and local health authorities also provide courses on super-vision. However, arguably the best way of learning how to do supervision is to experience it (Rowe, 2011).

Numerous models of supervision have been developed for mental health practitioners (see Bernard and Goodyear (2014) for an overview of models drawn from different disciplines). Different models may involve variations on aims, conceptual framework, and the roles and relationship of supervisor and supervisee. While it is not essential to use a model in supervision, it may help to guide you in thinking about the aims and focus of supervision. Models of super-vision often draw upon a particular area of theory, and it is important to under-stand the conceptual framework used, and choose a model that fits your area of practice (Sloan, 2006).

Conclusion

Supervision is a complex practice requiring care, skill and commitment. It is also a highly flexible practice, which can be modelled to suit your needs and aspi-rations, but this flexibility means that supervision can be in danger of becom-ing unfocused, muddled, unproductive and emotionally unsafe. It is therefore important before beginning supervision to ask yourself the key questions listed in the 'Activities' box.

Activities

Think about your responses to the following questions. Note down your answers if you find this helpful.

- Why do supervision?
  - What are my aims, motivations and expectations?
- With whom?
  - Who will my supervisor be?
  - What kind of supervision relationship do I want to have?
  - Will my supervisor also have supervision?
- How?
  - What will the focus of supervision be?
  - What do I *not* want to happen in supervision?
  - What will help me in my supervision practice (e.g. support of your tutor/employer, having allocated time for supervision)?
  - What will hinder me in my supervision practice (e.g. difficulty finding a supervisor)?
  - How will I know if supervision is working for me (e.g. agree a review process with your supervisor)?
- How will I deal with any problems in supervision?

Suggested reading

Bernard, J.M. and Goodyear, R.K. (2014) *Fundamentals of Clinical Supervision*, 5th edn. Boston, MA: Pearson.

Bond, M. and Holland, S. (2010) *Skills of Clinical Supervision for Nurses*, 2nd edn. Maidenhead: Open University Press.

Hawkins, P. and Shohet, R. (2012) *Supervision in the Helping Professions*, 4th edn. Maidenhead: Open University Press.

Each of these three books offers a comprehensive introduction to supervision in mental health care, covering theories and models of supervision, and practical considerations.

Shohet, R. (ed.) (2011) *Supervision as Transformation. A Passion for Learning*. London and Philadelphia: Jessica Kingsley Publishers.

A collection of personal accounts of having and giving supervision. This is a good book to read if you'd like to get a sense of what it feels like to have supervision.

The British Association for Counselling and Psychotherapy: www.bacp.co.uk

provides a list of accredited supervisors who are trained in counselling and psychotherapy supervision, but who are often willing to supervise members of other disciplines.

References

Bernard, J.M. and Goodyear, R.K. (2014) *Fundamentals of Clinical Supervision*, 5th edn. Boston, MA: Pearson.

Bradshaw, T., Butterworth, A. and Mairs, H. (2007) Does structured clinical supervision during psychosocial intervention education enhance outcome for mental health nurses and the service users they work with? *Journal of Psychiatric and Mental Health Nursing*, 14, 4–12.

Butterworth, A. (1992) Clinical supervision as an emerging idea in nursing, in Butterworth, A. and Faugier, J. (eds) *Clinical Supervision and Mentorship in Nursing*. London: Chapman and Hall.

Buus, N., Angel, S., Traynor, M. and Gonge, H. (2011) Psychiatric nursing staff members' reflections on participating in group-based clinical supervision: a semistructured interview study. *International Journal of Mental Health Nursing*, 20, 95–101.

Carroll, M. (2007) One more time: what is supervision? *Psychotherapy in Australia*, 13, 34–40.

Carroll, M. (2011) Supervision: a journey of lifelong learning, in Shohet, R. (ed.) *Supervision as Transformation. A Passion for Learning*. London and Philadelphia: Jessica Kingsley Publishers.

Cleary, M. and Freeman, A. (2005) The cultural realities of clinical supervision in an acute inpatient mental health setting. *Issues in Mental Health Nursing*, 26, 489–505.

Cleary, M., Horsfall, J. and Happell, B. (2010) Establishing clinical supervision in acute mental health inpatient units: acknowledging the challenges. *Issues in Mental Health Nursing*, 31, 525–531.

Clouder, L. and Sellars, J. (2004) Reflective practice and clinical supervision: an interprofessional perspective. *Journal of Advanced Nursing*, 46, 262–269.

Edwards, D., Burnard, P., Hannigan, B., Cooper, L., Adams, J., Jugessur, T., Fothergil, A. and Coyle, D. (2006) Clinical supervision and burnout: the influence of clinical supervision for community mental health nurses. *Journal of Clinical Nursing*, 15, 1007–1015.

Frawley-O'Dea, M.G. and Sarnat, J.E. (2001) *The Supervisory Relationship. A Contemporary Psychodynamic Approach*. New York: The Guilford Press.

Freshwater, D. (ed.) (2002) *Therapeutic Nursing: Improving Patient Care through Self-awareness and Reflection* [electronic resource]. London: Sage.

Frosh, S. (2012) *A Brief Introduction to Psychoanalytic Theory*. London: Palgrave Macmillan.

Gilbert, T. (2001) Reflective practice and clinical supervision: meticulous rituals of the confessional. *Journal of Advanced Nursing*, 36, 199–205.

Hawkins, P. and Shohet, R. (2012) *Supervision in the Helping Professions*, 4th edn. Maidenhead: Open University Press.

Hyrkäs, K. (2005) Clinical supervision, burnout, and job satisfaction among mental health and psychiatric nurses in Finland. *Issues in Mental Health Nursing*, 26, 531–556.

Hyrkäs, K., Appelqvist-Schmidlechner, K. and Oksa, L. (2003) Validating an instrument for clinical supervision using an expert panel. *International Journal of Nursing Studies*, 40, 619–625.

Johns, C. (2006) *Engaging Reflection in Practice. A Narrative Approach*. Oxford: Blackwell Publishing Ltd.

Jones, A. (1998) Clinical supervision with community Macmillan nurses: some theoretical suppositions and case work reports. *European Journal of Cancer Care*, 7, 63–69.

Koivu, A., Saarinen, P.I. and Hyrkäs, K. (2012) Does clinical supervision promote medical-surgical nurses' well-being at work? A quasi-experimental 4-year follow-up study. *Journal of Nursing Management*, 20, 401–413.

McLeod, J. (2013) *An Introduction to Counselling*, 5th edn. Maidenhead, Berkshire: Open University Press, McGraw-Hill Education.

Norman, I.J. and Ryrie, I. (eds) (2013) *The Art and Science of Mental Health Nursing: A Textbook of Principles and Practice*, 3rd edn. Maidenhead: Open University Press.

Playle, J.F. and Mullarkey, K. (1998) Parallel process in clinical supervision: enhancing learning and providing support. *Nurse Education Today*, 18, 558–566.

Proctor, B. (2001) Training for the Supervision Alliance Attitude, Skills and Intention, in Cutcliffe, J.R., Butterworth, T. and Proctor, B. (eds) *Fundamental Themes in Clinical Supervision*. London and New York: Routledge.

Rodgers, A. and Shohet, R. (2011) Supervision Through Conversation: Being Seen, Being Real, in Shohet, R. (ed.) *Supervision as Transformation. A Passion for Learning*. London and Philadelphia: Jessica Kingsley Publishers.

Rolfe, G., Freshwater, D. and Jasper, M. (2001) *Critical Reflection for Nursing and the Helping Professions. A User's Guide*. Basingstoke: Palgrave.

Rowe, A. (2011) 'It's at the heart of our practice in the Family Nurse Partnership Programme', in Shohet, R. (ed.) *Supervision as Transformation. A Passion for Learning*. London and Philadelphia: Jessica Kingsley Publishers.

Ryde, J. (2011) Supervising psychotherapists who work with asylum seekers and refugees: a space to reflect where feelings are unbearable, in Shohet, R. (ed.) *Supervision as Transformation. A Passion for Learning*. London and Philadelphia: Jessica Kingsley Publishers.

Schön, D.A. (1983) *The Reflective Practitioner*. London: Temple Smith.

Shohet, R. (ed.) (2011) *Supervision as Transformation. A Passion for Learning*. London and Philadelphia: Jessica Kingsley Publishers.

Sloan, G. (2006) *Clinical Supervision in Mental Health Nursing*. Chichester: John Wiley.

Stevenson, C. and Jackson, B. (2000) Egalitarian consultation meetings: an alternative to received wisdom about clinical supervision in psychiatric nursing practice. *Journal of Psychiatric and Mental Health Nursing*, 7, 491–504.

Todd, G. and Freshwater, D. (1999) Clinical supervision. Reflective practice and guided discovery: clinical supervision. *British Journal of Nursing*, 8, 1383–1389.

White, E. and Winstanley, J. (2010) A randomised controlled trial of clinical supervision: selected findings from a novel Australian attempt to establish the evidence base for causal relationships with quality of care and patient outcomes, as an informed contribution to mental health nursing practice development. *Journal of Research in Nursing*, 15, 151–167.

Yegdich, T. (1999) Clinical supervision and managerial supervision: some historical and conceptual considerations. *Journal of Advanced Nursing*, 30, 1195–1204.

Part 2
Therapeutic skills

3

Person-centred counselling

Theo Stickley and Paul Cassedy

Introduction

In this chapter we give an overview of person-centred counselling. This briefly includes its historical and theoretical origins, but importantly some examples of what this might look like in practice. Mental health nurses may frequently use counselling skills, but they should not be regarded as counsellors without first having undergone some kind of counselling training. All mental health nurses could undergo some form of person-centred counselling skills training in order to learn core skills for practice, which could be included in their pre-registration education. Because of the position we take, we believe that person-centred counselling skills are the most important skills nurses need in order to practise effectively in mental health services. This book contains chapters about many kinds of important skills, but we think the skills that we introduce in this chapter are of the utmost importance because they are foundational. In other words, we think that, without person-centred counselling skills, mental health nursing is seriously impeded.

Learning objectives

After reading this chapter, you will:

- have greater understanding of the historical influence of person-centred counselling
- understand person-centred counselling theory and its relevance to mental health nursing practice
- be able to identify the specific person-centred skills that are essential for successful mental health nurse practice.

Everybody has interpersonal skills to some degree. However, in order to learn to advance those skills, it is useful to acknowledge we all have the potential to develop our interpersonal skills. By taking a humble position and being open to developing this aspect of yourself, you will have the opportunity for greater self-awareness and ultimately for developing improved mental health nursing skills.

We begin the chapter by looking at concepts of self and self-awareness, and identify the importance of these concepts in mental health nurse practice. We also discuss the concept of the 'deliberate use of self' and the nature of therapeutic relationships. Much of the theory section in this chapter is informed by the work of Carl Rogers (1902–1987) who is acknowledged as critical in the development of the humanistic psychology movement that emerged in the 1950s–1960s. His work has influenced the development of person-centred counselling. In this chapter we identify these skills in practice and emphasise how intrinsic they are to successful mental health nursing.

Background to this approach

There are different ways of viewing the relationship we develop with service users. Humanistic psychology emerged in the second half of the last century and has sometimes been referred to as a 'third wave' (the first wave was psychoanalysis; the second was behaviourism). It is important therefore to identify what differentiates humanistic psychology from its predecessors. Both psychoanalytical thinking and behaviourism conceptualise people as victims of events and circumstances. Methods of therapy for both of these approaches involve an expert professional using their knowledge and training to help the victim come to terms with their psychological distress. Humanistic psychology has a very different focus. People are seen as basically good and each of us has the capacity for personal growth towards self-actualisation. What is important for this process to be successful is for each person to receive love and to have a sense of belonging. Once these foundations are established in people's lives, then they will flourish. In his book, *A Way of Being* (Rogers, 1980), Carl Rogers talks about when he was young, seeing a sack of potatoes that had been left in a basement. The shoots of the potatoes had grown '2 or 3 feet in length as they reached toward the distant light of the window' (p. 118). The shoots would never grow into healthy plants because they did not have the right conditions to flourish. Given the right conditions (soil, sunlight, water) they would grow into healthy plants and bear fruit. He likened human potential to the potential of the potatoes. Given the right conditions, humans can flourish and grow, and each of us has that innate tendency.

It is easy to understand this basic principle in relation to child development. It makes intuitive sense that children need unconditional love and acceptance, and to feel a sense of belonging in order for them to develop successfully. What Rogers did was to take one step further in applying this principle to helping relationships. While psychoanalysis and behaviourism used experts to treat service users, humanistic approaches require the therapist (counsellor or nurse) to unconditionally accept the service user, no matter what they are like or what they have done. Furthermore, it is important for the therapist to not judge the person. This, Rogers believed, would provide a *therapeutic relationship* and it is through this relationship that people can grow and change. This is of course asking a great deal of a therapist. It is relatively easy to imagine asking a parent to unconditionally love their child, but it is less easy to show love to a complete stranger, especially someone who may be quite unlikeable and might have committed offences. This example of person-centred theory raises, again, the need for self-awareness. It is extremely complicated to be asked to show love towards somebody you possibly do not like, and this is further complicated by having to be non-judgemental about somebody you may disapprove of. Nevertheless, this is what person-centred practice demands. A good discussion of these issues can be found in Stickley and Freshwater (2002).

We believe Carl Rogers was responsible for a major shift in the attitudes and practices of therapists, becoming aware of power differences in their relationships with service users, and moving from a directive approach to a non-directive, and thus person-centred, approach. It was in the 1970s and early 1980s that the person-centred culture began to have an impact on mental health services in the UK. As large institutions were being phased out and community care established, skills of promoting more independent living and choice making were needed, enabling people to develop their own inner resources and maintain a state of psychological well-being.

Concepts of self and self-awareness

Rogers contributed much to the concept of self. Prior to the 1950s, the greatest influences on the concept of self were arguably religion, psychoanalysis and behaviourism. Rogers' conceptualisation of self has become adopted into mainstream language today – for example, self-image and self-esteem. He also talks about an ideal self against which we judge ourselves, and this judgement determines our self-worth.

Our concept of ourselves is of course greatly influenced by our upbringing. If parents (and/or significant others) accept a child unconditionally, show unconditional love, and provide emotional security and physical safety, there is every chance the child will have a more secure sense of their own identity in later life. We might say that this child will grow up having a positive self-image and positive self-worth. Obviously this is an over-simplification and any number of circumstances might disrupt this process.

A key to understanding person-centred theory is to grasp the notion of 'unconditional love', or – as Rogers referred to it in his books – 'unconditional positive regard' in the context of therapeutic relationships. If a parent's love for a child is not unconditional, the child may believe they have to act in certain ways to please the parent (in order to receive the love that is needed). In these circumstances, the love of the parent then becomes 'conditional' rather than unconditional. When conditions are fixed by parents, the child will gradually develop what Rogers referred to as 'conditions of worth'. Instead, therefore, of a healthy and positive self-image, children may then experience a reduction in their self-esteem, because they are seemingly unable to please their parents without having to meet certain conditions of behaviour. A child may eventually enter adulthood without realising how, all through their childhood, their personality (and their self-image) has developed strongly influenced by the 'conditions of worth' they developed during childhood. Such a negative self-image can subsequently cause problems in later life.

Self-awareness, therefore, is a process of understanding these complexities within ourselves. It is one thing reading about such things in a textbook, but quite another to develop understanding about ourselves. Person-centred counselling therefore helps to promote self-awareness. The role of the counsellor is to provide unconditional positive regard in the counselling relationship, in order to create the right kind of conditions for trust to exist in the relationship. Once trust is established, the service user may begin the process of talking about themselves and the counselling relationship becomes established. Much of Rogers' work illustrates the nature of this relationship. He identified what he called 'core conditions' for a therapeutic relationship. In summary these are genuineness, non-judgemental acceptance and empathy. These all need to be provided by the counsellor. While this may sound like a simple formula, it is in fact an immensely complicated demand. These qualities require a great deal of self-awareness from the counsellor. That is why we assert that, in order to become a person-centred counsellor, it is necessary to undergo professional training. It is possible, however, to learn some basic skills to use in mental health nursing practice without having to undergo professional counselling training. We will illustrate some of these skills in the rest of this chapter.

Self-awareness in practice

Self-awareness is so much more than simply knowing about our likes, dislikes and preferences in life. Mental health nurses especially are required to develop self-awareness throughout their careers. This may mean some uncomfortable experiences. We need to be able to be aware of our beliefs, our values and our prejudices, and (most difficult of all) that there is much about ourselves we do not know. Our journey in mental health nurse education and practice also needs to be a journey into ourselves. Here is a short list of ways to develop self-awareness:

- listening to what others say about us
- inviting feedback from others about our practice
- keeping a reflective journal
- attending group or individual supervision
- attending personal counselling.

Developing self-awareness cannot happen quickly. It is mostly about our own personal and internal processes, and genuine, positive change will usually take quite a long time. This is true of ourselves and equally true about people with whom we work.

Integrating qualities and skills for a therapeutic session

Most of us will know how it feels when we have been in hospital, had an appointment at a health centre, or have been to see someone for help, advice and information. There are feelings of anxiety and apprehension, fear, and perhaps even humiliation. These typical feelings, when we are in a new situation and environment, can be because there is an imbalance of power in the relationship. The nurse in this situation has authority and control, and the other – the service user – does not. A first task for the nurse when engaging in and beginning a therapeutic relationship is to reduce this imbalance as much as possible. We may not have control over the location where the session takes place, but first impressions are of considerable importance to the service user. Mearns and Thorne (2007) say that power games can be played as much with tables and chairs as with words and tone of voice. The terminology of 'tables and chairs' can also refer to other obstacles and artefacts, clinical or otherwise, that give a message of power imbalance. We may not be able to remove the reception desk or other formalities of the environment, however, by reflecting fundamental humanistic concerns with relationship building and levelling power balances, we can make sure our seating arrangements, when having a session with a service user, convey equality, warmth and respect, and cause no (or very limited) distractions. A principle of person-centred interactions is to create equality in the relationship, where power is shared, and where authority and control over the service user are discarded. This means we also need to be aware of any clutter we may be bringing to the session, such as pens, keys or other clinical paraphernalia, which may cause a distraction. This could be physical as well as psychological – for example, any preconceived ideas we may have, intrusive outside thoughts or other trivial things on our minds. We must be able to offer our free and full attention (Casemore, 2011).

There will be many opportunities to talk with a service user in a person-centred way. One scenario to consider is presented in Box 3.1.

Box 3.1 Taking opportunities to be service user-centred

You may have noticed that Jo (a service user on a ward) looks preoccupied, anxious or sad. Her body language is different from usual and her tone of voice is rather flat. Your observations suggest that Jo looks worried, however you are not sure and, more importantly, Jo may not wish to talk at the moment. However, there is an opportunity to invite Jo to talk. This may be approached as follows:

You don't seem your usual self today, Jo. I'm wondering if there is something troubling you. Are you OK?

This offers respect to Jo, while indicating your concern, as you are not assuming there is something wrong. There is unlikely to be any threat to Jo to disclose personal thoughts or feelings, however there is an invitation to talk. This can be viewed as making an indirect enquiry as to her well-being.

In Box 3.2, the importance of structuring time and support is illustrated.

Box 3.2 Taking opportunities to structure time and support

Unlike with Jo (see Box 3.1), with other service users time and support can be more formal and therefore a more direct approach can be used. A first consideration is to structure the boundaries of time – as busy nurses we always seem to have time constraints (and so may the service user). We need to negotiate the time boundary together, for example:

Let's see, I have around 45 minutes at the moment, do you?

A more formal session may begin with:

I have an hour that we can spend together. Where would you like to begin?

Other opening statements might include:

How would you like to use the time we have together right now?

When you're ready, please feel free to start.

It is important to keep one's promise of the time boundary, as if not we may lose the trust of the service user. They may think that we are too busy to help, or they may feel unimportant or rejected, and that we do not value their worth, which perhaps for many is a familiar feeling. Keeping to a time boundary also maintains the professionalism of that particular therapeutic encounter, in that it will help separate this from the clinical or social interactions a nurse may have with a service user.

At the very beginning of the session we need to put the service user at ease; friendly smiles, gestures and introductions will enable this. Use of first names and using their name during the interaction will make the session more personal to that person. We need to be aware of our non-verbal communication skills, which indicate active and attentive listening, such as having an open and relaxed body posture, appropriate eye contact, nods, and appropriate head and arm gestures that convey warmth, respect and genuineness. It is best to maintain an unhurried pace that expresses we have time, and can give the person a sense of freedom to express themselves and *room to breathe*. As the session is *their* agenda, in terms of what they want to discuss and share, we need to have no preconceived plan or structure as to what they should do or how they should go about it.

Very often a nurse is there to give advice, to problem solve or give some direction to the service user. However with a person-centred approach, the emphasis is on the service user finding their own ways forward, trusting their innate tendencies for personal growth and development. This may be facilitated if the helper provides the necessary core conditions, as discussed earlier in this chapter. This approach may be unfamiliar to many of our service users, who at first may want, or expect, the nurse to take over and offer advice or opinion. This is illustrated in Box 3.3.

Box 3.3 Helping people to find their way forward

At the start of a session the service user may respond to the opening statement with:

Well I want your help and advice on …

or

I thought you could throw some light on this for me as to what is wrong.

A person-centred approach would reflect this back to the service user. For example:

Well, perhaps together we can come up with some ideas.

This indicates sharing of roles and responsibilities. Or:

Yes I can see you are having difficulties at the moment [indicates empathy]. *I would like to help* [indicates willingness], *so let's both of us explore what's going on?*

As we begin dialogue with the person, we are building and developing the quality of the therapeutic relationship, which to most, if not all, therapists is at the heart of their work and is central to successful interventions. We all tend to communicate and interact with people more successfully when we feel a connection or affiliation with them. To enable this with our service users, we need to develop a rapport. Rapport can be described as a harmonious understanding with another person, someone with whom we get on well. Having a connection with a person may happen naturally, but often this will need to be built and developed. Empathic relationship building, by our desire to connect with the person, will help develop rapport. This is illustrated in Box 3.4.

Box 3.4 Empathic relationship building

For example, ask the person if they could:

Tell me a little bit more about that?

Or:

I would like to understand more. What was that like for you?

Use clarification. For example:

I want to make sure I understand. Have I got this right ... ?

Focusing on the person and not the problem, and focusing on their experiences (which are likely to be different from our perceptions), will help you see much more of their viewpoint. By adopting an accepting manner, by communicating respect with a non-judgemental approach, we will also be laying foundations for the ongoing therapeutic relationship. We need to remain unshocked, by being aware of the messages we may be giving to the service user, such as signs of disapproval or alarm at what they are saying, as this can reinforce any anxiety or shame they might feel, in particular when talking about delicate or sensitive issues. Our approach needs to be unrushed, and should allow the person to talk at a pace they feel safe with. Consider who is doing most of the talking in the helping relationship. If we are asking service users to talk to us, or a person comes to us to talk through something, then that is what needs to happen. The service user talks and we listen. As helpers we need to feel comfortable with silence and lose the need to talk all the time. Silence can feel uncomfortable or even foolish. Come to make friends with silence. View it as working silence or therapeutic silence as we use it to fully concentrate and display attention to the service user. It is reflective time, time to pause for thought and clarity, and is valuable in facilitating the service user's own emotional processes.

Remember a service user-centred approach is not about trying to solve problems, but rather is about facilitating the person to talk freely and safely, exploring the issues that they feel are important, and to reach their own resolution.

Core skills of listening and responding

In this section we provide, in Box 3.5, a case study from practice to illustrate some of the core skills of a person-centred approach at work. There are two characters: Eden, the service user, and Maya, the mental health nurse. Eden is in his late twenties and has had two previous admissions to the mental health services. His father, who was a chronic alcoholic, died when Eden was 13. His mother suffers from depression. She has had numerous admissions to hospital, one of which followed a serious attempt on her life. Eden's elder sister joined the armed forces and had no further contact with the family. Eden left school with no qualifications, and has drifted in and out of casual employment. He has not experienced a nurturing relationship or a significant intimate relationship. He lives independently, although over the last three years his lifestyle has become more chaotic. He experiences anxiety when faced with decisions and has intruding thoughts that he is a worthless person. He gains some relief from excessive drinking and drug misuse, which often turn into crises for him. A recent self-harming incident resulted in a new admission. Previous psychiatric assessments have diagnosed schizo-affective disorder, personality disorder and drug-induced psychosis.

What follows in Box 3.5 is a short transcript of an encounter between the two people. Underneath the encounter we identify the skills that Maya is using as well as observe how Maya uses her person-centred approach for the benefit of the service user.

Box 3.5 Case study

Maya: Hello Eden. I've noticed today that you have not joined in so much ... you've been starting tasks and not completing them. I was wondering if there is something on your mind?

While offering a feedback statement on her observations, there is also an invitation to talk.

Eden: Yeah, suppose so. Not sure if I can fit in here and just worried about all sorts of stuff.

Maya: I'm sorry to hear that. Would talking to me about it help? I have time at the moment.

Shows interest and concern, along with a further invitation to talk.

Eden: If you think it might do some good?

Maya: I find talking to someone when I am worried helps.

By self-disclosing in a brief and purposeful manner, Maya begins to demonstrate genuineness in the relationship. They find somewhere quiet to sit, where they are unlikely to be disturbed. Maya adopts an open posture to demonstrate non-verbal listening skills (communicating warmth in the relationship).

Maya: You said earlier that you are not sure if this is the right place, and there are lots of things on your mind. Where would you like to start?

Maya paraphrases Eden's opening response, followed by an open question.

Eden: Well, life for me is in a bit of a mess right now. Can't seem to get my head sorted out with all that's going on.

Maya: All that's going on ...

Maya, reflects back Eden's last words – 'all that's going on' – which enables him to continue.

Eden: Can't hold down a job for long, behind with my rent, I know I shouldn't have drunk so much the other night, when I went off on one, now I regret it an' don't know what to do ...

Maya: You're feeling bad about what happened?

Maya makes an empathic reflection.

Eden: Guess so. Nothing good ever seems to happen for me.

Maya: Uh-huh.

Maya makes a minimal verbal prompt, along with non-verbal gesture of slight head nod, to keep the flow of the conversation going.

Eden: Not for long anyway. I seem to get things sorted out then everything gets shot down, and then I start to struggle, especially when decisions need to be made.

Maya: So you have had quite a few knockbacks. That must be difficult. Life seems a battle for you?

Paraphrasing and empathic response.

Eden: I get a knot in my stomach, tense up and all that, don't know what's going on in my head. It's difficult to explain.

Maya: Well, I think you're explaining it well, Eden. Go on.

Maya is affirming to Eden, communicates warmth and makes a minimal prompt for him to continue.

Eden: Do you? No one else seems to understand me, or even listens to me. They just tell me what I should or shouldn't be doing.

Maya: Who in particular tells you that?

Open question to help clarify.

Eden: Bosses I have worked for; a doctor I saw one time. They give me all this advice then I'm left to sort things out on my own. I get all in a muddle and confused.

Maya: That must be rather scary.

Empathic response.

Eden: It is.

[*There is some fear and then sadness in his eyes. He looks away from Maya*]

Maya remains silent with non-verbal attending, communicating warmth and that she is not going to leave Eden at this moment, and that it's OK to have these feelings.

Eden: Sorry about that. I'm pretty hopeless at expressing how I feel. Never good at nothing, that's me, was always told to shut up and not make a fuss.

Eden expresses conditions of worth.

Maya: You're doing OK. Feelings are often difficult to express, and often rather unnerving. You can express them to me.

Maya communicates genuineness, unconditional positive regard and offers support to Eden.

Eden: Yeah, perhaps maybe, I should get better at it.

Maya: Should?

Reflects back the word 'should', enabling Eden to continue.

Eden: Oh, I don't know. What do you think, you tell me?

Maya: [smiles] You don't seem to like other people telling you what you should do, now you're telling yourself what you should do. That must be confusing.

Maya avoids offering any kind of advice, instead offering a tentative challenge that may help Eden to clarify.

Eden: Guess so. Beat myself up, don't I? In all sorts of ways, like why I ended up in here.

Maya: It does sound like you give yourself a hard time, but now you are here and you have begun to talk, I feel I'm getting to know you better. You've been saying that although life at times has been OK, lately things have been going wrong: you lost your job and are behind with your rent. But perhaps more importantly at the moment, coping with problems is tough, you don't feel understood, or even understand yourself and your actions at times. Part of you is confused and you find that difficult to express. Would that be fair to say?

Maya offers warmth and genuineness, and then summarises the main aspects of their conversation.

Eden: Yes, more or less spot on. You seem to have understood me. I feel like you have listened to me.

Maya: [with a warm smile] Thanks. I appreciate you saying that.

Maya offers affirmation and genuineness.

The conversation could have continued and this will depend on time, resources and the type of treatment that is to be offered to Eden. The above encounter is an example of a person-centred interaction; it is only an example, though, and it could have taken several directions and focuses. However, it does follow certain principles of active listening skills in a person-centred context.

Maya uses mainly the following:

- **open questions** – generally requiring more than a one-word answer, invite the service user to expand further
- **minimal prompts** – encourage the service user to continue

- **reflecting key words** – mirrors back a key word the service user has said
- **empathic reflecting** – listens for and reflects back the feeling, which perhaps is not being voiced by the service user
- **paraphrasing** – rephrases succinctly and tentatively the essential and important content of what the service user has just said
- **self-disclosure** – used sparingly and appropriately, helps build rapport and deepen trust in the relationship
- **clarifying** – checks for understanding
- **therapeutic silence** – can help the service to gather their thoughts, conveys genuine interest, and allows time for deeper thoughts or feelings to emerge
- **affirmations** – the use of positive statements to the service user to affirm her/his value and importance as a human being
- **summarising** – the pulling together and restating of the key parts of the conversation as accurately as possible.

By using these skills Maya is communicating the qualities of warmth, genuineness and empathy. Her intention was to build a trusting relationship with Eden, where he would feel safe to express himself and be understood. She wanted him to feel valued and respected as a person; in this way she was communicating unconditional positive regard. By manifesting these core conditions in her relationship with Eden, and having faith and trust in his own capacity to grow, this would help restore and revitalise Eden's own belief in himself, reduce his conditions of worth and become a more fully functioning individual. Being valued and being able to value himself as a person would promote his ability to reach his potential, or to 'self-actualise'.

Maya helped Eden to explore his feelings and express them in constructive ways. He began to recognise some of his self-destructive tendencies and was able to work out for himself more positive ways of dealing with them. He began to feel more accepted and valued, aspects of himself he had never truly experienced before, which in turn helped his self-esteem and self-concept. By gradually enabling Eden to believe he was a person of worth he became more positive in his outlook towards himself and life in general.

Conclusion

Today there are many people who (although not working as psychotherapists and counsellors) use the ideas of Carl Rogers as guiding principles in their day-to-day work and relationships. This kind of approach is used widely by mental health nurses, and others such as teachers.

At one level, Rogers' theory and work are very simple to describe. As many people would attest, though – both those using this approach and those working as person-centred therapists/counsellors – they can be very difficult to put into practice because the approach does not use techniques but relies on the personal qualities of the therapist/person to build a non-judgemental and empathic relationship.

It could be argued that the British culture and indeed that of the mental health services, does not lend itself to a culture of a pure person-centred approach. There is competition among services, targets to meet, deadlines to keep. Perhaps the increase in intellectualisation and evidence-based practice has led to a decrease in reflecting on feelings and working at relational depth. We, however, continue to hope that a person-centred approach and culture will carry on growing among health care workers and mental health professionals. Helping people to find their own way in their recovery and problem solving enables the development of deeper levels of self-esteem and improved service user outcomes. When a person can recognise change has come about from their own actions, choices and decisions, this has a positive effect on their self-esteem, self-confidence and overall mental health.

One criticism of the person-centred approach, in its purest form, is that it lacks direction and structure, is too simplistic and can often end up going round in circles. Another viewpoint is that all therapists employ the core conditions in their work; we would like to think so. However the question is, are they just using these qualities while they are in the role of the helper or, as a genuine person-centred helper, take them fully on board and carry the spirit of them in all aspects of themselves and their lives? We would encourage all mental health nurses not only to learn person-centred theory, but to acquire genuine person-centred practice that comes from a core of person-centred values. In that way, we are far more likely to be able to effectively help the person with whom we are working.

Activity

Think about how person centred you are the next time you are in the practice area. Take time out to reflect on a time you have spent with a client. You might ask yourself some questions like those that follow, and write down your answers.

- How much of this interaction was focusing upon the professional agenda?
- How did I demonstrate to the client that I was listening?
- What feelings were aroused during this encounter?
- To what extent was I directive compared with being reflective?
- What would I improve upon if I were in a similar situation again?

You could share your reflections with your mentor or colleague.

Suggested reading

Norman, I.J. and Ryrie, I. (eds) (2013) *The Art and Science of Mental Health Nursing: A Textbook of Principles and Practice*, 3rd edn. Maidenhead: Open University Press.

There are two chapters in this book that would be helpful complementary reading for this chapter. Chapter 20, 'Counselling approaches', by Macchin and Westrip, offers an overview of the key principles of Carl Rogers' work and includes a useful section on ending counselling relationships. Chapter 12, by Ellis and Day, provides some ideas for qualities that help promote a therapeutic relationship and offers descriptions of the different kinds of therapeutic relationship that can exist.

Callaghan, P., Playle, J. and Cooper, L. (eds) (2009) *Mental Health Nursing Skills*. Oxford: Oxford University Press.

This edited book has chapters on interpersonal communication, values and caring.

References

Casemore, R. (2011) *Person-Centred Counselling in a Nutshell*, 2nd edn. London: Sage.

Mearns, D. and Thorne, B. (2007) *Person-Centred Counselling in Action*, 3rd edn. London: Sage.

Rogers, C. (1980) *A Way of Being*. Boston, MA: Houghton Mifflin.

Stickley, T. and Freshwater, D. (2002) The art of loving and the therapeutic relationship. *Nursing Inquiry*, 9, 4, 250–256.

4

Using a solution-focused approach

Nicola Evans

Introduction

Solution-focused therapy is just one of a number of therapeutic approaches that it might be helpful to adopt when working with people with mental health needs. As with other schools of therapeutic work, it is not simply a series of techniques, but is underpinned by a philosophy that guides the nature of the therapeutic relationship between the practitioner, or mental health nurse in this case, and the service user. This approach can be used in work with individuals, couples, families or groups to enable changes in behaviour or thinking. This chapter is intended to enable you to consider integrating some of the ideas from this therapeutic approach into your existing practice, and makes no claims to offer therapeutic training in this area. However, there is evidence that fundamental skills in using a solution-focused approach to therapeutic work can be acquired within a relatively short space of time and, once gained, can be effectively incorporated within a nurse's repertoire of therapeutic skills (Bowles, MacKintosh and Torn, 2001; Hosany, Wellman and Lowe, 2007; Ferraz and Wellman, 2009).

Solution-focused therapy originated from systemic family therapy (see Chapter 14). De Shazer (1985) is generally considered to be the founder of this approach. It is a model of brief therapy in which collaboration with the service user is fundamental, and therapeutic work is based around recognising the service user's strengths and building on them. Conversations using this approach are future focused, rather than trying to analyse what has happened before. In the explanation for this therapeutic approach, the service user would be advised that only a few meetings will be required, no more than five, and fewer if sufficient progress had been made. Due to the underpinning philosophy of this approach, solution-focused work can be used as either a single therapeutic approach or as an adjunct to other treatment modalities, depending upon the service user's needs and preferences.

Learning objectives

After reading this chapter, you will:

- have an understanding of the theoretical basis underpinning solution-focused therapeutic work
- be familiar with the assumptions underpinning a solution-focused approach to therapeutic work
- have been introduced to the main techniques used in a solution-focused approach to practice
- recognise opportunities in practice where adopting a solution-focused approach might be a useful intervention.

Theoretical basis of the solution-focused approach

Solution-focused brief therapy was developed by a team of family therapists at the Brief Family Therapy Center, Milwaukee, USA, in the early 1980s. This therapeutic approach is based upon taking a solution-building rather than a problem-solving approach to individuals, couples or families wanting change in their lives (De Shazer, 1985).

There are some assumptions made with this therapeutic approach that need to be understood and embraced. At its heart is the assumption that individuals are motivated to change aspects of their life, and this is evidenced by their actions to seek help. Other models (for example, cognitive behaviour therapy) may include in their therapeutic regimes strategies to increase or promote motivation for change, but in solution-focused work, this is accepted as implicitly present with the service users seeking assistance. Therapeutic work is considered within a collaborative framework between service user (or family) and practitioner. Collaborative care planning is a fundamental principle in mental health care in the UK currently but, within solution-focused work in particular, there is an assumption that there is equality within the therapeutic relationship. There is an inherent assumption within solution-focused therapy that all services users have existing strengths or resources. The role of the practitioner using this approach is therefore to enable the service user to draw on these resources to create a positive outcome for the service user in the context that, within this model, it is acknowledged that all service users have the potential for success (O'Connell, 2003).

One might argue that there are limitations to the fundamental assumptions underpinning solution-focused therapeutic work. For example, there are challenges in achieving an equal relationship with service users on occasion. People who are accessing help at a vulnerable point in their lives may be seeking an expert to help guide them, offer suggestions to improve their lives or give advice about a suitable course of action. If their mood is significantly low, or their thought processes impaired by poor concentration, it might be difficult for them to engage in this process of negotiation and discussion about how to identify and capitalise on the parts of their lives that are working effectively. Similarly, the definition of 'successful outcome' is open to a range of interpretations.

If we were to accept the underpinning assumptions of this model, however, and accept that by working collaboratively in an equal relationship with a service user who is motivated for change and has the potential for change, then we accept that a positive outcome is possible for the service user with this approach.

One of the strategies employed within this approach is the idea of locating exceptions. As we accept service users are best informed about their own lives, they are encouraged to recall occasions when they have overcome or successfully managed the difficulty or issue. These rare, or occasional, occurrences are known as exceptions and the service user can identify and draw on them. The final assumption is taken from systemic family therapy – it is the idea that even small changes in a person's life have the potential to create a big impact. A summary of the main assumptions of solution-focused therapy can be found in Box 4.1.

Using solution-focused approaches in mental health

There is evidence that solution-focused approaches are currently used in a variety of mental health settings and for multiple purposes. The approach has been used to inform mental health assessments (Ward, 2013), health promotion in mental health settings (Wand, 2011) and in inpatient services to promote service users' engagement with services (Bowles, Coughlan and Harnett, 2007). Coxon (2012) even suggests it is one of the core competencies that community mental health nurses should have.

Using solution-focused approaches across specialities

Solution-focused approaches have been found to be effective in helping people achieve behavioural change to improve their health. This has been reported in work with children (Nowicka, Pietrobelli and Flodmark, 2007; Reinehr et al., 2010) and adolescents (Nowicka et al., 2008) with weight gain problems, improving compliance for children with diabetes (Christie, 2008) and in decreasing substance use in adolescents (Froeschle, Smith and Ricard, 2007). Aside from direct clinical work, professional development (Fowler, 2011) and clinical supervision were areas where this therapeutic model also has application (Gupta and Woodman, 2010). Bond et al. (2013) conducted a systematic review of literature published in the English language between 1990 and 2010 that discussed solution-focused therapy with children and their families. They found that the evidence generally supported solution-focused brief therapy for this population, with more evidence to address issues where externalising behaviour was present in the children. They did suggest that further empirical studies were needed.

Box 4.1 summarises the assumptions underpinning solution-focused approaches.

Box 4.1 Summary of underpinning assumptions

- All service users are motivated
- Collaboration works
- Service users are best informed about their own life
- A positive outcome is possible
- Small changes have a big impact

Developing skills in the solution-focused approach

For ease of description, this therapeutic approach is described as if it were being offered on a sessional basis. This approach, however, also lends itself to a less formalised method of delivery, such as being incorporated within conversations that a nurse might have with a service user on a mental health ward, for example, or seeing a service user on a one-off basis if they present for triage, assessment or consultation at a mental health service.

As this is a brief therapeutic approach, the emphasis is on offering no more sessions than is absolutely required, with a range of between three and five sessions being common. For some people only one session is required to enable them to achieve sufficient change. For others, this approach might allow them to consider the options of longer-term treatment modalities. The frequency and duration of sessions are negotiated between the practitioner and service user. There is no assumption that sessions are an hour long, for example, or that they need to be on a weekly or monthly basis, although they could be if this would suit the service user. The overriding principle for the intervention is to do only as much as is required to enable the service user to move on with their life. Suggestions or interpretations of the service user's situation are only rarely offered and, if they are, are tentatively framed. The focus of collaborative talk between practitioner and service user is on the future, not the past, with the aim of achieving small changes that potentially create a big impact for the service user's life.

The five main steps in the therapeutic process are as follows:

1. problem identification
2. solution amplification – miracle questions
3. solution amplification – the use of scaling questions
4. solution amplification – locating exceptions
5. feedback.

To demonstrate solution-focused skills in action a hypothetical service user is used, introduced in Box 4.2.

Box 4.2 Introducing Heather

Heather is a 39-year-old woman, married with two sons. She has had a history of low mood/depression, which started following the birth of her second child, who has cerebral palsy. Heather attempted suicide through overdose three years ago and is currently accessing mental health services because her mood is low. She is currently on sick leave from work as a school administrative assistant. She is lying in bed much of the day, not sleeping well at night, rarely going out of the house and reports having no energy.

Step 1: problem identification

This is an opportunity for you to collaboratively explore with the service user what they would like to be better in their life. This may be the first time they have sought any therapeutic help, or it may be an opportunity for them to consider a different approach or to prioritise one specific aspect of their life. Using this approach you are interested in discovering with the service user why they are now seeking help for a specific issue. It may be that the service user has a multitude of worries. The initial collaboration would focus on helping them to identify their highest-priority goals and to select one that is achievable. It is important to acknowledge with the service user that they may have a number of issues, but that making a selection as to which one to focus on is in itself a useful strategy. This is demonstrated in Box 4.3, which illustrates this in the context of helping Heather.

Box 4.3 Problem identification

Practitioner: So, Heather, I am interested to know what has made you look for help at this stage?

Heather: My whole life is just so awful. My husband said I should come, he brought me, and the GP said the medication won't work on its own.

Practitioner: So, of all of your whole life that is awful, what aspects do you hope I could help with today?

Heather: I can't be bothered with my boys, I'm tired all the time, I feel awful, I can't even go to the shops to get the groceries ... there's so many things.

> *Practitioner:* You have mentioned a few parts of your life that you would like
> to be different. Of those that you have mentioned, which do you think
> you would say is your priority right now?
> *Heather:* I'm not being a very good mother to my boys, I never play games
> with them, or read with them, I feel so guilty. They must hate me or
> wish they had a different mother.
> *Practitioner:* So am I right in thinking, most of all what you would like is to
> be different in the way you respond to your sons right now?

During this process, the practitioner would look for an opportunity to identify an area where a small change would be achievable and have a positive impact for the service user, being transparent with the service user about the rationale. In the above example, this might be a small, achievable task that Heather could accomplish in relation to responding to her sons differently. This step would be followed by the development of a collaborative plan about what small area or issue the service user could target.

At this stage, it can also be useful to invite the service user to consider any pre-session change that has occurred in relation to their identified issue before they began the conversation today. This could simply be asked, as follows:

> *Practitioner:* What has changed about the way you respond to your sons
> since you decided to come here for help?

This would have the effect of reinforcing the positive aspects of any changes actually made independently, or if the service user responds that no change was made, the practitioner could observe that the service user has come for help, which is a step towards the service user's goal, thus empowering the service user.

Step 2: solution amplification – asking the miracle question

The miracle question (Box 4.4) is designed to allow the service user to think freely about the possibilities of this part of their life being different. It invites an optimistic or hopeful response. It encourages the service user to think playfully about options they would not normally consider. Service users are effectively being asked to imagine what an ideal or perfect solution might look like. Care needs to be taken in using the term 'miracle' question, though, as it may offend some cultural or religious groups, but in the literature on solution-focused therapy this is often how this question is defined. In addition to paying attention to the cultural context, miracle questions can be adapted to suit other contextual factors such as the age of the service user. If the service user were a child, different language might be used. I have sometimes used the term 'magic wishes' in its place. This technique is demonstrated in Box 4.4.

Box 4.4 Asking the miracle question

Practitioner: I am going to ask you a strange question now, but imagine a miracle happened overnight and, tomorrow, the way you are respond-ing to your boys is fantastic. What would that look like?

Heather: Imagine! I need a miracle! Well I'd be brilliant with them.

Practitioner: What would that look like, being brilliant with them?

Heather: We'd be laughing, I'd roll on the floor tickling them, we'd play football in the garden, I'd read them their favourite stories using funny voices.

Going through the miracle question process has allowed the service user to think of how life might be better in relation to that aspect of it that they have prioritised. This can then be used to identify and locate a small step in the general direction towards that improvement by using scaling questions.

By using a question about what the change would look like, the focus is on observable behavioural change, which can be noticed by both the service user and others.

Step 3: solution amplification – the use of scaling questions

This is a technique (see Box 4.5) for enabling the service user to consider realistic, achievable goals as stepping stones towards their miracle position. For this process the service user is asked to describe what a 100 per cent solution would be to the issue they want to be better in their life. They then would be asked to imagine what a 5 per cent step towards that goal might present to themselves or to others.

Box 4.5 Scaling

Practitioner: That sounds such good fun for them and you. Just imagine if you were to get 5 per cent towards being that brilliant, what would that look like? What do you think would your husband notice about the way that you and the boys are together?

Heather: I think if I were just that 5 per cent that you suggest, I think my husband would see me doing their reading homework with them when they just get home from school.

Step 4: solution amplification – locating exceptions

In this step (see Box 4.6) the practitioner helps the service user to recall or identify occasions when they have either managed to do what they wished, or their situation that represents the 5 per cent stage of the miracle outcome has been close to their ideal. This is then followed by an exploration of what the circumstances were around this exception to the current difficulty, and a dialogue about how replicating aspects of the circumstances surrounding the exception might be recreated. The dialogue in Box 4.6 illustrates one way of locating an exception.

Box 4.6 Exceptions

Practitioner: During the last few months, while you have been feeling 'awful', as I think you described, have there been any occasions when you have been able to do any reading with the boys?

Heather: No, I don't think so.

Practitioner: OK, so have you read half a page with either of them, or read a bedtime story to them?

Heather: Definitely not. I can't remember – it must be ages, apart from when Josh (my son) had to learn his lines for the school concert.

Practitioner: That must have been very important to you, to be able to help Josh to learn his lines for the concert even when you were feeling so awful. I wonder if it might be possible to try that again?

Heather: Well, I only spent five minutes with him each night for about a week. It wasn't much really.

Practitioner: But in fact you did spend five minutes each evening a few times a week, so whatever was happening was working for you. Let's try to think about that time in detail to work out how you did it.

Heather: Well, I had to help him learn his lines otherwise it would have been upsetting for him, not being able to join in the school concert.

Locating an exception and identifying with the service user an occasion where they were unexpectedly or uncharacteristically successful in the area they had identified as their priority allows the identification of some factors that contributed to that success, so they can be repeated. As Quick (1998) suggests, where an aspect of a service user's world is functioning well for them, encourage them to do more of that.

Step 5: feedback

This is the stage at the end of a session or a solution-focused conversation (see Box 4.7). The service user is invited to consider whether they would like some feedback on either the session or on homework they may have completed in between sessions.

If the service user declines the offer of feedback, they are commended on their engagement with the process and invited to continue to do more of what is working for them, and to notice how it is happening. The service user is also invited to stop doing anything that is unhelpful or that is not working.

If the service user would like feedback, validate the feelings they have expressed during the session. A genuine compliment about the service user's commitment to engage in the process will encourage further effort. There is also the opportunity to offer a suggestion or homework that the service user might do in the near future. After feedback, the service user is asked whether or not they would like a further session or conversation about this issue, or whether they would like to be signposted to another service, if relevant.

Box 4.7 Feedback

Practitioner: I understand how awful you have been feeling about not being able to give your sons as much attention as you have done in the past and I am genuinely impressed that despite feeling so tired, Heather, you are committed to doing something to change that. I wondered if you were able to find an opportunity just once this week to read with your son, whether you would be able to notice how you were feeling after you had done this?

At this stage, you and the service user agree whether or not a further conversation or session would be useful to the service user, remembering the guiding principle is that no more sessions than needed should be offered. In this therapeutic approach, booster sessions, or evaluation appointments, are not used.

Conclusion

A solution-focused approach can be a useful addition to a mental health nurse's toolkit. It is a brief therapeutic approach that builds on a service user's strengths. It can be used as a stand-alone intervention or in conjunction with other approaches. It is based on a collaborative approach with a service user, and uses the service user's strengths and knowledge about themselves to create an opportunity for change for the service user. The simple techniques of using a 'miracle question' or looking for an 'exception' can provide an opportunity when working therapeutically with a service user to think creatively and widely about possible alternatives that could help them to overcome their presenting obstacles.

The use of scaling helps a service user to consider achievable and measurable steps towards a complete solution. These steps reinforce a sense of moderation in planning for the service user. Being successful at making or identifying small steps encourages the service user to continue to strive for further gains, in a measured, stepwise way.

Activity

In order to develop your knowledge of this approach there are a number of useful publications, both books and journal articles, that give a good overview. The European Brief Therapy Association website has up-to-date information on conferences, and discussion about research and emerging practice in the field. You could also consider reflecting on a service user you have met, either on your own or in supervision, to consider whether this approach might be helpful for them. You may also be able to secure appropriate clinical supervision specifically to develop your skills in this area. You could discuss with a supervisor how using this approach might have been useful for a service user. If you are able to identify a supervisor to specifically help you develop these skills, discuss how you might rehearse these skills in a safe way and then attempt them under supervision. The use of audio-recorded material, with a service user's permission, is a good way to give you the opportunity to reflect on your own practice. You can accurately hear what was said and how to engage with the service user, and use this as material to either think how you might do things differently, or to take to a group or individual supervision session for external critique.

You may also have the opportunity to observe experienced practitioners using this approach in the field, or indeed be able to watch their video-recording of sessions, provided permission had been obtained beforehand from the service user to use this material for teaching purposes.

Suggested reading

The European Brief Therapy Association website can be accessed at www.ebta.nu. On this site you will find details of conferences and discussion about solution-focused work, as well as links to papers.

Hawkes, D. (1998) *Solution-focused Therapy: A Handbook for Healthcare Professionals.* Oxford: Butterworth-Heinemann.

This text was written by a mental health nurse who later trained in systemic therapy. He also has a useful chapter on using a solution-focused approach for people experiencing psychosis in:

O'Connell, B. and Palmer, S. (2003) *Handbook of Solution-focused Therapy.* London: Sage Publications.

References

Bond, C., Woods, K., Humphrey, N., Symes, W. and Green, L. (2013) Practitioner review: the effectiveness of solution focused brief therapy with children and families: a systematic and critical evaluation of the literature from 1990–2010. *Journal of Child Psychology and Psychiatry*, 54, 7, 707–723.

Bowles, N., Coughlan, A. and Harnett, P. (2007) Becoming solution focused in acute inpatient psychiatry wards, part 1: becoming solution focused. *Irish Nurse*, 8, 5, 16–17.

Bowles, N., MacKintosh, C. and Torn, A. (2001) Nurses' communication skills: an evaluation of the impact of solution-focused communication training. *Journal of Advanced Nursing*, 36, 3, 347–354.

Christie, D. (2008) Dancing with diabetes: brief therapy conversations with children, young people and families living with diabetes. *European Diabetes Nursing*, 5, 1, 28–32.

Coxon, G. (2012) Mental health competencies for practice and community nurses. *Nursing in Practice*, 64, 24–26.

De Shazer, S. (1985) *Keys to Solution in Brief Therapy*. New York: Norton.

Ferraz, H. and Wellman, H. (2009) The integration of solution-focused brief therapy principles in nursing: a literature review. *Journal of Psychiatric and Mental Health Nursing*, 15, 37–44.

Fowler, J. (2011) Supporting self and others: from staff nurse to nurse consultant, part 9: solution-focused support. *British Journal of Nursing*, 20, 17, 1138.

Froeschle, J.G., Smith, R.L. and Ricard, R. (2007) The efficacy of a systematic substance abuse programme for adolescent females. *Professional School Counselling*, 10, 5, 498–505.

Gupta, V. and Woodman, C. (2010) Managing stress in a palliative care team. *Paediatric Nursing*, 22, 10, 14–18.

Hosany, Z., Wellman, N. and Lowe, T. (2007) Fostering a culture of engagement: a pilot study of the outcomes of training mental health nurses working in two UK acute admission units in brief solution-focused therapy techniques. *Journal of Psychiatric and Mental Health Nursing*, 14, 688–695.

Nowicka, P., Pietrobelli, A. and Flodmark, C.E. (2007) Low-intensity family therapy intervention is useful in clinical setting to treat obese and extremely obese children. *International Journal of Paediatric Obesity*, 2, 4, 211–217.

Nowicka, P., Haglund, P., Pietrobelli, A., Lissau, I. and Flodmark, C.E. (2008) Family weight school treatment: 1-year results in obese adolescents. *International Journal of Paediatric Obesity*, 3, 3, 141–147.

O'Connell, B. (2003) Introduction to the solution-focused approach, in O'Connell, B., Palmer, S. (eds) *Handbook of Solution-Focused Therapy*. London: Sage Publications.

Quick, E. (1998) Doing what works in brief and intermittent therapy. *Journal of Mental Health*, 7, 5, 527–533.

Reinehr, T., Kleber, M., Lass, N. and Toschke, A.M. (2010) Body mass index patterns over 5 years in obese children motivated to participate in a 1 year lifestyle intervention: age as a predictor of long term success. *American Journal of Clinical Nutrition*, 91, 1165–1171.

Wand, T. (2011) Real mental health promotion requires a reorientation of nursing education, practice and research. *Journal of Psychiatric and Mental Health Nursing*, 18, 2, 131–138.

Ward, T. (2013) Positioning mental health nursing practice within a positive health paradigm. *International Journal of Mental Health Nursing*, 22, 2, 116–124.

5

Motivational interviewing

Michelle Huws-Thomas

Introduction

One of the biggest challenges that mental health nurses face is helping people deal with entrenched patterns of behaviour that impact upon engagement in treatment and recovery. Lack of motivation, loss of interest in everyday activities, poor adherence to prescribed pharmacotherapies, and neglected lifestyle behaviours are common factors in people suffering with moderate to severe mental distress that lead to relapse and further deterioration in mental and physical health (DiClemente, Nidecker and Bellack, 2008). These patterns can be frustrating to mental health nurses in the face of carefully delivered case formulations and goal planning, engendering frustration and lost hope. Research around behaviour change shows that motivation is a dynamic state that can be influenced in response to a practitioner's style of communication (Rollnick, Miller and Butler, 2008; Hall, Gibbie and Lubman, 2012). This chapter focuses on motivational interviewing (MI) (Miller and Rollnick, 2002, 2013) as an appealing psychological counselling approach, arguably because it is non-confrontational, with the onus on empowerment being in the hands of the individuals themselves. While the holy grail of finding the specific elements that are most effective in the practice of MI have yet to be identified (Apodaca and Longbaugh, 2009), researchers are beginning to explore the active ingredients that practitioners seek in dealing with everyday consultations with people who use their services. Specific skills will be discussed that the mental health nurse can draw upon in their practice.

Learning objectives

After reading this chapter, you will:

- understand the background and theoretical basis of MI

- recognise some mental health conditions in which MI has been demonstrated to be effective
- be able to explore the phases and specific skills required to practise MI
- be able to reflect on practice challenges and ongoing skills proficiency in MI.

Background to motivational interviewing

Motivational Interviewing (MI) is defined as:

> a collaborative, goal-oriented style of communication with particular attention to the language of change. It is designed to strengthen personal motivation for and commitment to a specific goal by eliciting and exploring the person's own reasons for change within an atmosphere of acceptance and compassion.
>
> (Miller and Rollnick, 2013, p. 29)

Motivational interviewing may be described as an evolution of the person-centred therapy developed by Carl Rogers (1957), who emphasised empathic understanding of the service user's frame of reference and therapist communication style as the core relational conditions for service user growth and change (Westra and Aviram, 2013; see also Chapter 3 in this book). A conversation where the mental health professional engages the individual in a dialogue that is service user centred, and explores the discrepancy between the person's most deeply held values and their current behaviour, is more likely to be successful than when the mental health professional argues or instructs for change to occur (Miller and Rollnick, 2002).

While MI lacks a coherent theoretical framework, there are many theoretical influences contributing to the factors within the method. Miller (1983), for example, described MI as being based on principles of experimental social psychology, drawing on principles of cognitive dissonance theory (Festinger, 1957), psychological reactance theory (Brehm, 1966), self-efficacy (Bandura, 1977) and the Stages of Change Model (or Transtheoretical Model, TTM) (Prochaska and DiClemente, 1983).

MI also has roots in the behaviourist tradition and integrates elements of service user-centred therapy with behaviour therapy whereby the mental health nurse values people for who they are, while helping them identify ways in which they would like to change and develop plans to make those changes (Wagner and Ingersoll, 2013). Miller and Rose (2009) proposed an emerging theory of MI that emphasised two specific active components: a *relational* component focused on empathy and the interpersonal spirit of MI, and a *technical* component involving the evocation and reinforcement of service user change talk – formerly known as self-motivational statements (Miller and Rollnick, 2002).

Ambivalence is a central concept in MI and assumes that individuals will often vary in their degree of motivation to engage in treatment or look after themselves in health-affirming ways (Rollnick, Mason and Butler, 1999). Honouring this ambivalence and personal autonomy in decision making is achieved through the 'spirit' of MI, which emphasises a 'working with' rather than a nurse-led style of communication, whereby the individual appraises and reflects upon their internal conflicts and values that impact upon their short- and longer-term goals (Miller and Rollnick, 2013).

Motivational interviewing for mental and physical health problems

While MI was initially developed to help service users overcome problems relating to substance misuse, the evidence base is expanding to its effectiveness with people experiencing a wide range of mental and physical health problems (Arkowitz et al., 2008). Motivational Interviewing may be delivered as a stand-alone treatment for service users experiencing mild to moderate mental health distress, or as an adjunct to more intensive cognitive behaviour therapy (CBT), which can facilitate the engagement of service users with complex mental health problems in treatment (Hettema, Steele and Miller, 2005; Hides et al., 2010). Preliminary research supports the effectiveness of MI with service users experiencing a range of mental health problems, including substance misuse (Smedslund et al., 2011), anxiety (Slagle and Gray, 2007), depression (Westra, 2004), suicidality (Zerler, 2009), obsessive compulsive disorder (Simpson and Zuckoff, 2011), non-adherence to anti-depressants (Interian et al., 2010; Balán, Moyers and Lewis-Fernández, 2013) and binge eating (Dunn, Neighbors and Larimer, 2006; Vella-Zarb et al., 2015), and in increasing awareness to address problematic behaviours in PTSD-related difficulties (Murphy, 2002). An integrated MI–CBT intervention has demonstrated promise in resolving ambivalence about substance misuse for individuals experiencing bipolar disorder and co-morbid substance misuse problems (Jones et al., 2011).

Mental health nurses are well placed to deliver MI either as a brief intervention of between one and four individual sessions (each lasting typically 45–60 minutes), as an adjunct to existing treatments such as CBT (Westra, Aviram and Doell, 2011), within groups (Wagner and Ingersoll, 2013) or adapted in conjunction with other treatments, whereby minor adaptations (known as AMIs) refer to specific techniques the mental health nurse can draw upon in their practice. Box 5.1 summarises some of the key features of the MI approach.

Box 5.1 Key features of motivational interviewing

Motivational interviewing (MI) is a popular psychological counselling approach among mental health nurses due to the non-confrontational approach and emphasis on individual empowerment. The evidence base is expanding to show its effectiveness with individuals experiencing a wide range of mental and physical health problems.

Most MI interventions have been effective as an adjunct to other psychological therapies, such as cognitive behaviour therapy (CBT).

How MI fits into mental health nursing practice

Motivational interviewing has been identified as an ideal therapeutic approach for managing complex mental health issues within clinical practice (Westra and Arkowitz, 2011). Miller and Rollnick (2002, 2013) proposed two phases. During the initial phase, intrinsic motivation for change is elicited by examining and resolving ambivalence, enhancing the importance of change and bolstering self-efficacy. The second phase is designed to strengthen the service user's commitment to change by considering change options, setting goals and making plans. Progression from the first to the second phase of the intervention is determined by the individual's readiness to change.

Core skills

Phase 1: rapport building and building motivation for change

The initial stage for the mental health nurse is to engage the person by developing rapport using Rogerian techniques, to identify problematic behaviour(s) and current concerns, and to elicit the service user's motivations for change. Within this phase, MI includes four key principles and three communication styles. The four key principles are as follows.

1. **Express empathy:** seeing the world through the person's eyes.

2. **Support self-efficacy:** to support the person in his/her belief that change is possible.

3. **Roll with resistance:** statements demonstrating resistance are not challenged.

4. **Develop discrepancy:** motivation for change occurs when a person perceives a discrepancy between where they are and where they want to be.

The three communication styles deemed important in behaviour change conversations are: (1) *guiding* (encouragement); (2) *directing* (signposting); and (3) *following* (supporting). Examples of these in action appear below. Motivational interviewing focuses mainly on *guiding* the person to want to change their behaviour, but all three styles may be used within the therapeutic dialogue, depending on the relationship between the mental health nurse and the service user, and the context (setting) of the dialogue (Miller and Rollnick, 2013).

Case study of MI in practice
In Box 5.2 you have the opportunity to meet Heléne, as a precursor to learning more about MI in practice.

> ### Box 5.2 Case study
>
> Heléne Wiseman is a 22-year-old university student who has been referred to the community mental health team (CMHT) with a nine-month history of depression and panic. She has lost more than 8 kilos over the past six months, isolates herself in her student house and is binge drinking up to a bottle of wine each night to help her sleep. Heléne is reluctant to be assessed as she has been prescribed anti-depressants from her GP in the past, which she says didn't help, and she found adhering to low-intensity CBT (Improving Access to Psychological Therapies) counselling difficult. While she says she wants to feel better, she isn't hopeful that the mental health nurse within the CMHT can help her. She feels distressed at the thought of having to practise exposure-based techniques again, which involve engaging in activities that are anxiety provoking, and learning to manage this.

Assessment and rapport building
The first task is to engage Heléne in treatment, establish a rapport and help explore the key areas of her life that most concern her. While assessment may be an important part of the overall treatment this can often place the individual in a passive role if conducted in a dialogue that is expert led and with an emphasis on psychiatric diagnoses. Indeed, Miller and Rollnick (2013) argued that assessment feedback is not an essential part of MI, although the authors recognise it may be useful in enhancing motivation in those experiencing lower readiness to change. The goal for the mental health nurse is to listen carefully and offer reflective listening statements, which are fundamental for mutual understanding. Miller and Rollnick (2013, p. 62) suggest that one of the most fundamental skills in MI, both in engaging the person and during MI sessions, is demonstrated in the acronym OARS: asking **O**pen questions, **A**ffirming, **R**eflecting and **S**ummarising. It has been suggested that the emphasis should be on reflections rather than repeated open questions in the ratio 2:1. Affirmations validate and show respect for efforts and strengths, and are most effective when they target a specific effort or strength (Naar-King and Suarez, 2012). Reflections are high-level skills in MI that are key in accurate listening and supporting the person in the discussion about change (Skinner *et al.*, 2013).

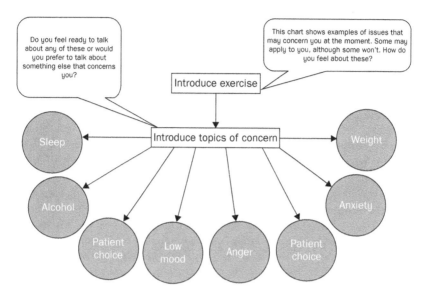

Figure 5.1 Example of agenda mapping

Agenda mapping

Agenda mapping (see Figure 5.1) is a key component of MI, and offers an opportunity for the mental health nurse and person to select a behaviour (or a selection
of problematic behaviours) that cause(s) most concern for the person (Miller and
Rollnick, 2013). Heléne's priorities for change may alter as sessions develop (e.g.
she may wish to focus more on her social isolation rather than her ongoing anxiety) as she develops greater awareness and self-efficacy. It is useful to refer to the
agenda map at the start of each prospective session as a reference point. Options
are to support Heléne to choose the topics of focus (or to introduce new ones), and
to offer (from a practitioner viewpoint) difficult subject areas as priorities, such as
eating issues or drinking that threatens her health. Importantly the agenda-setting
map is completed in a service user-centred spirit that preserves her autonomy.

Building the service user's motivation for change

The four principles of MI

The initial focus is to build Heléne's motivation for change using the four key
principles of MI: (1) reflective listening and acceptance (e.g. 'You are worried
about trying exposure therapy due to your past experience; it is not unusual
for people experiencing panic to be in two minds, what we call ambivalence,
about starting therapy'); (2) developing discrepancy between Heléne's current
and ideal situation (e.g. 'You currently feel depressed and you are isolating yourself, although on the other hand you want to feel "alive" again'); (3) rolling with
resistance (e.g. 'Nothing much has worked for you up to now'); and (4) building

self-efficacy in the belief she can carry out the necessary actions and succeed in changing (e.g. 'You managed to attend the IAPT workshops and, while you found it difficult, you succeeded in getting there').

The expression of empathy is fundamental and any dialogue about changing Heléne's behaviour will be accepted only when she feels personally valued.

Possible therapeutic dialogue

> *Mental health nurse:* You mentioned earlier you feel totally stuck. In order for me to get a sense of your difficulties, would it be OK to talk about your sadness and isolation and how it makes you feel? [*permission seeking*]
>
> *Heléne:* Well, yes I avoid everyone and feel really down, although I am worried about how much I drink and my panic attacks. [*note that Heléne's priorities are drinking, and her panic and sadness vs the practitioner's priorities of depression and isolation; the mental health nurse switches focus to her concerns about drinking and how it helps her cope, placing an emphasis on personal choice and changing direction*]
>
> *Mental health nurse:* Your drinking and anxiety concern you more than your isolation from friends and family? [*open-ended question*]
>
> *Heléne:* Absolutely. I am dying a slow death with my drinking. It helps me forget things, albeit for a while.
>
> *Mental health nurse:* Although it helps you forget your worries, it also concerns you. [*reflective statement*]
>
> *Heléne:* I am drinking so much that I worry I will get thrown out of university and then that will be the end for me.
>
> *Mental health nurse:* You worry that your drinking will end your studies and can't see how you might carry on if that happened. [*reflective statement*]
>
> *Heléne:* Well, I feel trapped because, on the one hand, I drink because I am so panicky and sad, and yet I am aware that it might ruin everything for me [*statement of ambivalence*]. I know that carrying on the way I am isn't helpful to me. I am not sure how you can help me.

Within the above dialogue, the mental health nurse's task is to help Heléne explore and articulate her key concerns, and to focus on what is most valued to her. Having established a therapeutic relationship and engaged Heléne in a helpful conversation about her key concerns, the next step is to focus on her possible discrepancy in changing her behaviour.

Evoking motivation for change
Now that a therapeutic relationship has been established and Heléne is engaged, the next step is evoking motivation for change (Miller and Rollnick, 2013).

Evoking change talk
Eliciting change talk is key to eliciting the individual's motivations and providing a way to resolve their ambivalence (Miller and Rollnick, 2013). The DARN acronym

(Desire, Ability, Reasons, Need) can help the mental health nurse generate open questions that elicit change talk in addition to more generic questions.

- **Desire:** 'What do you want, wish for, hope, etc.?'
- **Ability:** 'What can or could you do to make that change?'
- **Reasons:** 'What would be beneficial about changing?', 'How are these behaviours impacting on you?'
- **Need:** 'How important is it for you to change?'

Exploring ambivalence

Ambivalence is a type of resistance that occurs within the individual and reflects competing motivational forces, such as, 'There is a part of me that knows I need and want to change, and yet another part of me that stops me from changing.' This can be seen in Heléne's response 'on the one hand I drink because I am so panicky and sad, and yet I am aware that it might ruin everything for me'. Exploring ambivalence helps guide the individual to a satisfactory resolution of conflicting motivations (Miller and Rollnick, 2013).

A common decisional tool is the use of a ruler on an imaginary scale of 0–10. Rollnick, Miller and Butler (2008) advised that the most productive questions to explore within the decisional ruler are those to do with the importance of change and confidence in making a change. Within Heléne's consultation a mental health nurse might explore her values around importance and confidence as follows.

Exploring importance

On a scale of 0–10, where 0 is 'not at all important' and 10 means 'the most important thing for me right now', how important would you say it is for you to cut down on your drinking?

The value for change talk can be explored with a follow-up question:

You say you are at 6 and not 3 (or a lower number). Could you tell more me about this number?

Exploring confidence

Confidence is important. If the commitment to a change is low and Heléne has little confidence in her ability to change, then it is essential to continue with MI-consistent strategies until importance increases.

Decisional balance: pros and cons

Another popular way of exploring ambivalence within MI is a decisional balance exercise (see Table 5.1), which elicits the pros and cons (advantages vs disadvantages) of current behaviour. In the case of the consultation with Heléne, the exercise may help raise her awareness of her inner conflict about the cons of her current behaviour, which far outweigh the pros (or vice versa).

Table 5.1 Pros and cons decisional balance

Good things about my sadness	Not so good things about my sadness
I don't have to go out and socialise	I feel dreadful most of the time
I can avoid university	I worry I will fail my degree
My friends look after me	I drink to help cope with my low mood
I don't have to try to look after myself	I get panicky in lots of situations I want a boyfriend, which is impossible right now My drinking is making me skint My parents and friends are all worried about me
Good things about making a change	Not so good things about making a change
I will feel better	I will continue to feel awful
I will be able to cope with university better	I will need to give up drinking
My parents and friends won't feel so worried	I will need to try really hard
I can get back to my usual bubbly self	I am not confident I can do it
I can maybe get a boyfriend and go travelling	
I can socialise again	
I can start taking care of myself again	

Table 5.1 shows that the pros far outweigh the cons, which paves the way for further exploration about Heléne's motivation for change by evoking change talk. It may be, however, that having reached a decision about change Heléne will still experience inner conflict, which can be resolved through further exploration of the discrepancy between her goals and values. If the pros and cons are equal, Heléne may still reach a decision about change despite her ambivalence. Either way, the focus is on intrinsic motivation to change through empathy, reflective listening, building self-efficacy and rolling with resistance. The ultimate goal is for the individual to make her or his own decision about change rather than being coerced.

Phase 2: the how of change – planning and goal setting

The focus in this second phase shifts to strengthening the commitment to change, and supporting the individual to develop and implement a plan to make changes. Miller and Rollnick (2013, p. 257) suggest that, 'whilst the move to planning is a judgement call, the service user you are working with will tell you'.

Table 5.2 Change plan

What are my goals?	Cut down on my drinking Attend university lectures Take care of myself better Go out with my friends once a week
The most important reasons I want to change are	To not feel depressed and panicky To feel well again To get my degree
Things I can do to help me towards my goal	Listen to/read my mindfulness CD/book Go swimming Attend lectures on time Tell my mum when I feel down
How others can help support me in my goals	*Mum*: phone me daily to check on me *Friend Lisa*: Text me to prompt me to go swimming
I know my plan is working if	I am feeling less sad I am having contact with friends and family I feel less panicky

There are four parts to developing a change plan: setting goals, considering change options, arriving at a plan and eliciting commitment (Miller and Rollnick, 2013). Table 5.2 outlines a change plan that Heléne might develop with the mental health nurse. While Heléne may be committed to reducing her drinking, she may still feel ambivalent about seeing the mental health nurse on an ongoing basis. A change plan can be developed that focuses on reducing Heléne's drinking, attending university, being in contact with family and friends, and improving her self-care. The key point is that the plan is developed by Heléne herself.

Box 5.3 further summarises key features of the MI approach.

Box 5.3 Further key features of motivational interviewing

The overall style of MI is *guiding*, which lies between and incorporates elements of directing and following styles.

Motivational interviewing focuses more on service user perspectives than on framing issues from a practitioner perspective.

Ambivalence is a normal part of preparing for change and a place where a person can remain stuck for some time.

Change tends to occur when an individual perceives a discrepancy between important values and their current (often undesired) behaviour.

Conclusion

Motivational interviewing is a collaborative conversational style for strengthening a person's own motivation and commitment to change. MI proposes *two phases*: the first is concerned with eliciting the intrinsic motivation for change, and the second is designed to strengthen the service user's commitment to change. The evidence base for MI as an effective intervention outside substance misuse is growing and mental health nurses are well placed to deliver MI in practice. How a practitioner communicates with an individual can substantially influence intrinsic motivation. MI includes four key principles – (1) express empathy, (2) support self-efficacy, (3) roll with resistance, and (4) develop discrepancy – and three communication styles: (1) guiding; (2) directing; and (3) following. Overcoming obstacles through personal reflection and supervision is key to avoiding common traps in the therapeutic dialogue.

Activities

Activity 1
Think about a service user in clinical practice that you find 'challenging'. This may be a person who demonstrates a reluctance to talk about a specific issue or a person for whom nothing seems to be changing. You may think about a specific person or identify a hypothetical scenario.

- Reflect on what thoughts and feelings are evoked in you.
- How might you work collaboratively in practising the MI method with this person? Use the ideas and techniques from this chapter to frame your response to this.

Activity 2
How will you ensure proficiency in your MI skills in clinical practice? Think about your ongoing practice, supervision and follow-up coaching. What method(s) work best for you?

Suggested reading

Arkowitz, H., Westra, H.A., Miller, W.R. and Rollnick, S. (2008) *Motivational Interviewing in the Treatment of Psychological Problems*. New York: Guilford Press.

An edited book introducing the use of MI with people with a wide range of difficulties.

Mason, P. and Butler, C.C. (2010) *Health Behaviour Change: A Guide for Practitioners*, 2nd edn. London: Churchill Livingstone.

An accessible, practical book aimed at health practitioners and students.

Miller, W.R. and Rollnick, S. (2013) *Motivational Interviewing, Helping People Change*, 3rd edn. New York: Guilford Press.
This book serves as the complete introduction to MI.

Websites

Professor Stephen Rollnick: www.stephenrollnick.com
The website of an MI founding figure.
Motivational interviewing website: www.motivationalinterview.org
Provides details on how to find a MINT supervisor, international training, conferences and bibliographies.
MI-campus: www.mi-campus.com
Describes itself as a gateway for learners and practitioners in MI.

References

Apodaca, T.R. and Longbaugh, R. (2009) Mechanisms of change in motivational interviewing: a review and preliminary evaluation of the evidence. *Addiction*, 104, 5, 705–715.

Arkowitz, H., Westra, H.A., Miller, W.R. and Rollnick, S. (2008) *Motivational Interviewing in the Treatment of Psychological Problems*. New York: Guilford Press.

Balán, I.C., Moyers, T. and Lewis-Fernández, R. (2013) Motivational pharmacotherapy: combining motivational interviewing and antidepressant therapy to improve treatment adherence. *Psychiatry*, 76, 3, 203–209.

Bandura, A. (1977) Self-efficacy: towards a unifying theory of behavioural change. *Psychology Review*, 84, 191–215.

Brehm, J.W. (1966) *A Theory of Psychological Reactance*. New York: Academic Press.

DiClemente, C.C., Nidecker, M. and Bellack, A.S. (2008) Motivation and the stages of change among individuals with severe mental illness and substance abuse disorders. *Journal of Substance Abuse Treatment*, 34, 1, 25–35.

Dunn, E., Neighbors, C. and Larimer, M.E. (2006) Motivational enhancement therapy and self-help treatment for binge eaters. *Psychology of Addictive Behaviors*, 20, 1, 44–52.

Festinger, L. (1957) *A Theory of Cognitive Dissonance*. Stanford, CA: Stanford University Press.

Hall, K., Gibbie, T. and Lubman, D.I. (2012) Motivational interviewing techniques: facilitating behaviour change in the general practice setting. *Australian Family Physician*, 41, 9, 660–667.

Hettema, J., Steele, J. and Miller, W.J. (2005) Motivational interviewing. *Annual Review of Clinical Psychology*, 1, 91–111.

Hides, L., Carroll, S., Lubman, D.I. and Baker, A. (2010) Brief motivational interviewing for depression and anxiety, in Bennett-Levy, J., Richards, D.A., Farrand, P., Christensen, H., Griffiths, K.M., Kavanagh, D.J., Klein, B., Lau, M.A., Proudfoot, J., Ritterband, L., White, J. and Williams, C. (eds) *Oxford Guide to Low Intensity CBT Interventions* (pp.177–185). Oxford: Oxford University Press.

Interian, A., Martinez, I., Iglesias Rios, L., Krejci, J. and Guarnaccia, P.J. (2010) Adaptation of motivational interviewing interventions to improve anti-depressant adherence among Latinos. *Cultural Diversity and Ethnic Minority Psychology*, 16, 2, 215–225.

Jones, S., Barrowclough, C., Allott, R., Day, C., Earnshaw, P. and Wilson, I. (2011) Integrated motivational interviewing and cognitive behaviour therapy for bipolar disorder with comorbid substance misuse. *Clinical Psychology and Psychiatry*, 18, 426–437.

Miller, W.R. (1983) Motivational interviewing with problem drinkers. *Behavioural Psychotherapy*, 11, 147–172.

Miller, W.R. and Rollnick, S. (2002) *Motivational Interviewing. Preparing People for Change*, 2nd edn. New York: Guilford Press.

Miller, W.R. and Rollnick, S. (2013) *Motivational Interviewing: Helping People Change*, 3rd edn. New York: Guilford Press.

Miller, W.R. and Rose, G.S. (2009) Toward a theory of motivational Interviewing. *American Psychologist*, 64, 6, 527–537.

Murphy, R. (2002) Development of a group treatment for enhancing motivation to change PTSD symptoms. *Cognitive and Behaviour Practice*, 9, 4, 308–316.

Naar-King, S. and Suarez, M. (2012) *Motivational Interviewing with Adolescents and Young Adults (Applications of Motivational Interviewing)*. New York: Guilford Press.

Prochaska, J.O. and DiClemente, C.C. (1983) *The Transtheoretical Approach: Crossing Traditional Boundaries of Therapy*. Illinois: Dow/Jones Irwin.

Rogers, C.R. (1957) The necessary and sufficient conditions of therapeutic personality change. *Journal of Consulting Psychology*, 21, 95–103.

Rollnick, S., Mason, P. and Butler, C.C. (1999) *Behaviour Change: A Guide for Practitioners*. London: Churchill Livingstone.

Rollnick, S., Miller, W.R. and Butler, C.C. (2008) *Motivational Interviewing in Health Care: Helping Patients Change Behaviour (Applications of Motivational Interviewing)*. New York: Guilford Press.

Simpson, H.B. and Zuckoff, A. (2011) Using motivational interviewing to enhance treatment outcome in people with obsessive-compulsive disorder. *Cognitive and Behavioural Practice*, 18, 1, 28–37.

Skinner, W., Cooper, C., Ravitz, P. and Maunder, R. (2013) *Motivational Interviewing for Concurrent Disorders*. New York: W.W. Norton.

Slagle, D.M. and Gray, M.J. (2007) The utility of motivational interviewing as an adjunct to exposure therapy in the treatment of anxiety disorders. *Professional Psychology: Research and Practice*, 38, 4, 329–337.

Smedslund, G., Berg, R.C., Hammerstrøm, K.T., Steiro, A., Leiknes, K.A., Dahl, H.M. and Karlsen, K. (2011) Motivational interviewing for substance abuse. *The Cochrane Database of Systematic Reviews*. Chichester: Wiley. Online at www.thecochranelibrary.com (accessed 19 August 2014).

Vella-Zarb, R., Westra, H.A., Carter, J.C. and Keating, L. (2015) A randomized controlled trial of motivational interviewing + self-help versus psychoeducation + self-help for binge eating. *International Journal of Eating Disorders*, 48, 3, 326–332.

Wagner, C.C. and Ingersoll, C.S. (2013) *Motivational Interviewing in Groups (Applications of Motivational Interviewing)*. New York: Guilford Press.

Westra, H.A. (2004) Managing resistance in cognitive behavioural therapy: the application of motivational interviewing in mixed anxiety and depression. *Cognitive Behaviour Therapy*, 33, 4, 161–175.

Westra, H.A. and Arkowitz, H. (2011) Integrating motivational interviewing with cognitive behavioural therapy for a range of mental health problems. *Cognitive and Behavioural Practice*, 18, 1–4.

Westra, H.A. and Aviram, A. (2013) Core skills in motivational interviewing. *Psychotherapy*, 50, 3, 273–278.

Westra, H.A., Aviram, A. and Doell, F.K. (2011) Extending motivational interviewing to the treatment of major mental health problems: current directions and evidence. *Canadian Journal of Psychiatry*, 56, 11, 643–650.

Zerler, H. (2009) Motivational interviewing in the assessment and management of suicidality. *Journal of Clinical Psychology*, 65, 11, 1207–1217.

6
Using the skills of problem solving
Steven Pryjmachuk

Introduction

It is essential that mental health practitioners are skilled in problem solving because mental health practice is fundamentally about finding solutions to problems. In this chapter, we explore the 'theory' and 'practice' of problem solving by, first, considering what a problem is, and then examining some of the various models and techniques available that might help you and the service users you work with to problem solve. Following this, we explore problem solving in action, using one specific problem-solving model – the nursing process – as a framework for examining how practitioners might work with service users in identifying, crystallising and solving the sorts of problems that are typical in mental health practice. We also touch on the associated interpersonal, communication, assessment, interviewing and reflective skills that are necessary if you are to be an effective problem solver or, better still, effective in supporting service users to solve their own problems.

Learning objectives

After reading this chapter, you will:

- appreciate that problem solving is primarily a process that involves different stages
- have explored several problem-solving models and techniques
- have considered the importance of associated interpersonal, communication and therapeutic skills when problem solving in mental health practice
- have had an opportunity to see how problem solving can work in practice using the nursing process as a specific framework.

Theoretical basis

As its name suggests, problem solving is a specific type of thinking (a specific cognitive process) concerned with finding solutions to problems. The word 'problem' can have a variety of meanings, all of which allude to a difficulty of some sort that needs to be overcome. Box 6.1 contains definitions from the online version of the *Oxford English Dictionary*.

On first sight, only one of these four definitions (or problem types) – matters or situations regarded as unwelcome, harmful, or wrong – seems relevant to mental health practice. It could be argued, however, that mental health practitioners are also exposed to the other three problem types in their day-to-day practice. Theoretical psychiatry is, after all, driven by difficult and demanding questions like 'What causes schizophrenia?' (or even 'Does schizophrenia exist?'), 'Are mental illness and creativity connected?' and 'Are mentally disordered offenders mad or bad?' Technically, these difficult and demanding questions are known as *uncertainties* (Han, Klein and Arora, 2011) but they are, in reality, nothing more than what might be termed 'grand' problems. Psychiatry and mental health practice, moreover, often throw up puzzles and enigmas such as why some people recover completely from a single episode of schizophrenia while the majority do not (Rosen and Garety, 2005), or why electro-convulsive therapy, a controversial and poorly understood treatment (Anderson and Fergusson, 2013), seems to help some people. Even mathematical propositions are relevant when drug calculations are considered. Problem-solving skills are thus essential if you are to be an effective mental health practitioner.

Box 6.1 Defining 'problem' (*OED Online*, 2013)

A 'problem' is:

- a puzzle or riddle or enigmatic statement;
- a difficult or demanding question;
- a matter or situation regarded as unwelcome, harmful, or wrong;
- a mathematical or scientific proposition requiring that something be done.

In order to be skilled at problem solving, however, you need to understand the various ways in which problems can be solved. Perhaps the best known is *trial-and-error*, a method in which a potential solution is tried out and eliminated if it does not work, only to be followed by another potential solution, and so on. Trial-and-error can work in relatively simple, practical settings where there are a limited number of potential solutions (the assembly of flat-pack furniture without printed instructions, for example), though it can be somewhat time consuming. The utility of trial-and-error methods in mental health practice is limited, however. Of much greater value are what might be termed 'scientific' methods of problem solving. These methods are based around *rules*, whether these rules are explicit and rigid, or whether they are implicit and flexible. Where the rules are explicit and rigid, the methods are termed *algorithmic*; where they are implicit and flexible, they are termed *heuristic*.

As their name implies, algorithmic methods employ *algorithms*, which are explicit rules for specific tasks or situations. Examples of algorithms include the step-by-step instructions of computer programs, mathematical formulae, flow charts and decision trees. Algorithmic methods of problem solving are useful where there is a 'right' solution, such as calculating a drug dose or knowing what to do when someone absconds from a ward (the algorithm here being an absconding, or 'AWOL', procedure).

Heuristic methods of problem solving, on the other hand, can be conceptualised by terms such as *common sense, intuition* and *rule-of-thumb*. They are methods that draw upon a person's knowledge and experience, and are likely to be the most useful to you when problem solving with service users. Heuristic problem-solving techniques work well when there is no obvious solution, or no single 'right' solution. Hunches, sudden insight and past experiences of success can all drive heuristic problem solving in that they can provide the foundations of potential solutions, whether those potential solutions are conceived individually or more collaboratively. Indeed, in group problem-solving settings, the very point of activities like *brainstorming* or *action learning sets* (see Lamont, Brunero and Russell, 2010) is to force these hunches, insights and past experiences into the open so that viable, potential solutions can be identified.

At this point, you might think that putting potential solutions (whether conceived individually or collaboratively) into practice and evaluating their relative success sounds a bit like trial-and-error but in heuristic problem solving there are two subtle differences. First, the potential solutions that are trialled are not arbitrary; they are based on heuristics (common sense, intuition, rules of thumb, etc.) and, in collaborative settings, consensus. Second, as you will soon discover, there is a feedback loop so that any 'errors' (failures), and indeed successes, can be reflected upon, analysed and used to guide further potential solutions.

Specific problem-solving models

A variety of heuristic problem-solving models exist, many of which have been developed in business settings (where problem solving is also important). For example, one widely used business problem-solving model is PDCA (**P**lan–**D**o–Check–Act). PDCA was developed in the 1940s by the physicist Walter A. Shewart and, being a cyclical process, it is also known as the Shewhart Cycle or, alternatively, as the Deming Cycle after William A. Deming who popularised the model (Best and Neuhauser, 2006). Figure 6.1 summarises the elements of PDCA. Examining Figure 6.1, you will see that potential solutions to the problem emerge from the 'Plan' stage, 'Do' is the trial stage, 'Check' the evaluative stage and 'Act' the feedback loop to the initial 'Plan' stage.

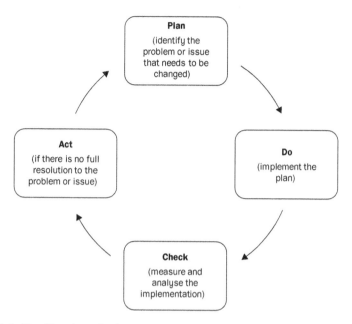

Figure 6.1 The Shewhart Cycle

Other well-known problem-solving models include GROW (see Whitmore, 2009; discussed in a related context later in this chapter), Eight Disciplines, or 8D (see Rimbaud, 2011), and How to Solve It (Pólya, 1957).

The nursing process

Another problem-solving model – and the one perhaps most useful for mental health practitioners – is the *nursing process*. The nursing process is usually seen as a cycle with four stages: assessment, planning, implementation and evaluation. However, Pryjmachuk (2011) argues that the leap from assessment to planning requires an interim stage where assessment results are crystallised to guide planning and that, since the process is cyclical and since evaluation can be seen as 'reassessment', assessment and evaluation are essentially one and the same (see Figure 6.2).

Those of you reading this chapter who are not nurses should not be put off by it being called the *nursing* process because, as McKenna (1997) points out, it is a process that all health care professionals can employ. Indeed, while the stage between assessment and planning is termed 'specific problem identification', it also amounts to what psychiatrists might call a 'diagnosis' or what psychologists might call a 'formulation'. You might also want to think about the similarities between the nursing process and the PDCA model.

Box 6.2 summarises this section's key points.

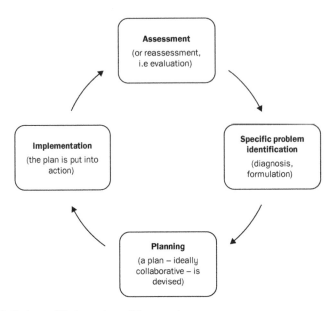

Figure 6.2 A modified version of the nursing process
Source: after Pryjmachuk (2011)

Box 6.2 Section key points

- A problem is a difficulty of some sort that needs to be overcome.
- Problem solving can be seen as a process that involves a series of discrete stages.
- There are many problem-solving models and methodologies around that can help you to work through the process.
- The nursing process is an ideal framework for helping you understand problem solving in mental health practice.

Problem-solving skills in action

Any of the problem-solving models outlined above – or indeed from other sources – can be used to frame problem-solving work in mental health practice. However, because of its general utility, and the fact it is a relatively straightforward model, we will explore problem-solving skills in action by considering each stage of Pryjmachuk's version of the nursing process in turn.

Assessment: identify the problem

The key to identifying the problem is a comprehensive *assessment* of the service user. Assessment has been considered in detail in Chapter 1 so we will not dwell on it here other than to reinforce a few important points and caveats regarding assessment. First, there is a whole variety of assessment tools and frameworks around, including formal diagnostic tools like the Structured Clinical Interview for DSM-IV (SCID; First *et al.*, 1996), those based on nursing models such as Orem's Self Care Model (see Orem, 2001) or the Tidal Model (see Barker and Buchanan-Barker, 2005), and more localised mental health assessments such as the Manchester Care Assessment Schedule (MANCAS; see Firth, 1999). What assessment tools you end up using is likely to be down to a combination of professional preferences, your own personal choice and the demands of the service in which you are working.

Second, a necessary prerequisite for conducting assessments is the possession of sound interpersonal and communication skills (Callaghan, Playle and Cooper, 2009; Pryjmachuk, 2011). It is important to maintain eye contact, rapport and a natural level of conversation with service users during assessment, but also important to ensure that the assessment is comprehensive, i.e. that nothing important has been left out. With beginners, there is often a tendency to over-focus on the assessment tools at the expense of maintaining a natural conversation or, alternatively, a tendency to concentrate so much on maintaining a natural conversation that important information is missed. So long as you are aware of these tendencies, you do not need to worry too much as the more opportunities you get to practise, the more skilled you will become. If you watch experienced, expert mental health practitioners undertake assessments, you will observe rapport, eye contact and natural conversation to the extent that the assessment becomes secondary and almost intuitive, and the practitioner seems to need a printed assessment tool merely as a prompt. But if you were to check their written notes afterwards, you would find that not only has the conversation been natural, they will have elicited every bit of important and relevant information needed to work with the service user. It is also important to *listen* to what the service user is saying and to not draw inferences without checking the accuracy of any such inference. Consider the dialogue in Box 6.3, taken from an initial assessment.

Box 6.3 Listening and drawing accurate inferences

Person seeking help: I feel so low since my girlfriend left me; everything seems so grey and empty. I wonder whether things will ever get better and sometimes think, 'If only I didn't wake up, would anyone care?' Funny mentioning waking up because if only I got some sleep, I might feel a bit better. I am absolutely exhausted by it all.

Naive practitioner: OK, so it's clear to me that your problem is depression. [*or, worse, the practitioner deems the person seeking help to be a suicide risk without probing things further with them*]

> Compare this with an expert practitioner . . .
>
> *Expert practitioner:* OK, so you're telling me you're feeling low, but con-
> nected to all of this is the trouble you're having sleeping. Is sleep
> perhaps your main problem at the moment? Tell me more about your
> sleep patterns.

This does not preclude investigating whether there is a potential suicide risk or not – indeed, risk assessment is a key element of comprehensive assessment in mental health – it is just that the expert practitioner has clearly understood that there is more to feeling low than a diagnosis of depression, encouraging the service user to agree or disagree with the suggestion that sleep might be the main problem at this point.

Specific problem identification: crystallise the problem

The second part of the process is to crystallise the problem as a *diagnosis* or a *formulation*. It was mentioned earlier that different mental health practition-ers have different preferences here, but Carey and Pilgrim (2010) argue that, since formulations are less stigmatising than diagnoses and since diagnoses have a tendency to ignore the causes of, or provide an explanation for, someone's psychological distress, formulations better serve the needs of service users and should thus be the preferred option.

According to the British Psychological Society's Division for Clinical Psy-chology (2011, p. 2), a formulation 'can be understood as both an event and a process'. The *process* of formulation requires a consideration of a broad range of biopsychosocial factors (identified during the assessment process), and it requires personal meaning and collaboration between servicer users and practi-tioners. The formulation *event* is an agreement (usually in written form) on the shared perspective of service user and practitioner. Box 6.4 gives an example of a (spoken) formulation proposed by an expert practitioner, which would usually be written down once agreed with the service user.

Box 6.4 Formulation

> *Expert practitioner:* So, let me just check: you've been feeling particularly
> down since your girlfriend left you; you've lost all interest in the things
> you used to like doing – football, going to the pub and socialising with
> your mates. You're feeling really tired because intrusive thoughts keep
> you awake most nights and this is having an impact on your work to the

> point that you feel you could be in trouble at work. This worries you, but not to the point that you would do anything to harm yourself though you don't know what you will do if you don't start feeling better soon. The key problem for you at the moment is not being able to sleep. You feel that, if you could sleep, you might be able to get into a frame of mind where you could start to think about things more rationally.
> Do you think I've summarised your position well? Is there anything you disagree with?

Indeed, depending on the service user's capabilities, you might even get them to propose the formulation in the first instance.

Planning: identify potential solutions

Clearly, potential solutions need to be linked to the identified (and agreed) problem, but sometimes it can also be helpful to explore what the particular *goals* of the service user are if it is not explicit in the formulation. Goal setting is explored elsewhere in this book, but is worth mentioning here that there are several goal-setting frameworks around (again drawn mainly from business settings) that you might find useful when working with service users – for example, SMART and GROW.

'SMART' goals (see Doran, 1981) are goals that are **S**pecific, **M**easurable, **A**chievable, **R**ealistic and **T**ime-bound. An example of a SMART goal is given in Box 6.5.

Box 6.5 Example of a SMART goal

To have a largely uninterrupted sleep of at least five hours a night most nights over the next week.

- Specific – it is a clear statement
- Measurable – 'five hours a night most nights' in a one-week period
- Achievable – seven hours might be unrealistic at the moment
- Realistic – as above
- Time-bound – a time ('over the next week') is specified

'GROW' (see Whitmore, 2009) is also an acronym, with the letters standing for, respectively, **G**oal, **R**eality, **O**ptions and **W**ay forward. GROW is a coaching as well as a problem-solving framework and, since Shepherd, Boardman and Slade (2008) argue that mental health practice is often akin to coaching, GROW has some value in mental health practice. As with SMART goal setting, the 'Goal' element of GROW requires that a specific goal is established in collaboration with the person being coached (or service user being supported). 'Reality' involves checking whether the goal is realistic. This can help the person being coached to identify any obstacles to achieving the goal. 'Options' is concerned with how any such obstacles might be dealt with in order to devise a 'Way forward' – an action plan – to achieve the goal.

Potential solutions to any identified problems can be elicited in a variety of ways. As we discussed earlier, techniques such as brainstorming and action learning sets can be useful in group settings; in one-to-one situations, creative problem-solving techniques such as *lateral thinking* (de Bono, 1970) or *mind-mapping* (Buzan and Buzan, 2009) might also be helpful. In any case, it is important that the service user is facilitated to find their own potential solutions. This not only ensures that the process is *collaborative*, it also helps the service user evaluate their own internal and external resources and so can help in building *resilience*. Moreover, it ensures that practitioners are operating within a philosophy of *recovery-focused care* by supporting service users to take control and responsibility for their own lives (Shepherd *et al.*, 2008).

Box 6.6 presents an example of how you might go about eliciting a range of potential solutions in a *collaborative* way.

Box 6.6 Eliciting solutions in collaborative style

Expert practitioner: What do you think I can do to help you sleep? ... And what do you think you can do yourself to help with sleep?

Person seeking help: I dunno. I've looked on the internet and I could take sleeping tablets, but that just seems too easy and people say they stop working after a while. What do you think?

Note that any response you give to service users must be *evidence based*. Compare the naive practitioner response in Box 6.7 with that of the expert practitioner.

Box 6.7 The importance of evidence

Naive practitioner: Yes, good idea. I'll arrange some sleeping tablets from your GP. I am sure they will help.

Expert practitioner: OK, well, yes you are right – the evidence shows that sleeping tablets can work, but they are only really a short-term solution and some can be addictive. It sounds like you'd prefer to try an alternative. Is that right? There are some other methods around that we can talk about and maybe you could give them a try. If they don't work, or things get worse, you could always come back to see me or your GP and then think about whether sleeping tablets might be a reasonable short-term option.

Implementation: test the potential solutions

In the implementation stage, potential solutions are tested (trialled) simply by asking the service user to try them out. While this can be relatively straightforward, it is often more complicated because mental health problems often adversely affect motivation and/or elicit scepticism in service users. A lack of motivation, for example, is common in depression and is present in 'avolition', one of the so-called 'negative symptoms' in psychosis. While *motivational interviewing* (see Chapter 5) and *behavioural activation* (see Chapter 11) may be useful here, it is the interpersonal and communication skills of the practitioner that will be paramount in helping the service user overcome his or her lack of motivation. In particular, you might use your skills to break down any actions into a number of smaller steps. This of course ties in with our earlier discussion of setting (SMART or GROW) goals that are both achievable and realistic. Consider the dialogue in Box 6.8 as an example of these skills in action.

Box 6.8 Testing solutions

Expert practitioner: So, we've agreed that when you said you 'used' to like football, you really meant you want to like it again but it doesn't have the appeal it once had; you think it won't be fun and your mates won't want you hanging around. How about going to watch your mates play Sunday football as a first step?

Person seeking help: I'm not sure. They won't want me near them and I won't have the energy and I'll be tired, and I'll just be worried they'll all be talking about me.

Expert practitioner: Mmm, so you've just given me every reason for not going to Sunday football! How do you know that all of these things will happen if you don't test them? And, remember, all that stuff about exercise being good for you and improving your mental well-being isn't just made up – there's good scientific evidence for it. Why don't you just *try* going and see how it goes before you write it off completely?

Reassessment: evaluate its success

The final step in the process is evaluation, or reassessment. Here the practitioner discusses the relative success, or otherwise, of any potential solutions they have tried. If a potential solution has not worked then the situation should be reassessed with the service user and alternative actions devised. Indeed, skilled practitioners often negotiate with service users a range of alternative solutions as contingencies. *Reflective skills* (see Chapter 2, or Rolfe, Jasper and Freshwater, 2010) are also useful in this stage, for both practitioner and service user. For the practitioner, reflection on the relative success or otherwise of any suggestions they may have made can help them improve future practice in that the practitioner will have tacit evidence for what might or might not work with service users with similar problems. For the service user, reflection can help them build resilience by identifying particular strategies and resources that might help them cope in the future.

When assessing the relative success or otherwise of any potential solution, be careful of *cognitive biases* that can influence the worldview of service users. *Confirmation bias*, for example – whereby people look for information to confirm their worldview – is extremely common. Can you see the confirmation bias in Box 6.9? How might you respond to it?

Box 6.9 Confirmation bias

Person seeking help: I've just had a text to say they can't go out with me tonight as their daughter is ill; I told you no one liked me.

Box 6.10 summarises key points from this section.

Box 6.10 Section key points

- A comprehensive assessment is the key to identifying problems
- Problem solving requires high levels of interpersonal and communication skills on the part of the practitioner
- Problem solving works best when it is collaborative
- Collaborative formulations are a good way of crystallising the problem
- Reflection on the relative success, or otherwise, of potential solutions can be beneficial to both service user and practitioner

Conclusion

The aim of this chapter is to introduce you to the concept of problem solving, discuss its value to, and use in, mental health practice, and to explore the underpinning skills required to problem solve. Now, at the end of the chapter, it should be clear to you that problem solving is an essential component of effective mental health practice, that problem solving can be at its most effective when truly collaborative and when framed by systematic processes like the nursing process, and that a comprehensive assessment of the service user is an intrinsic part of the problem-solving process. Moreover, underpinning the problem-solving process is the need for high levels of interpersonal and therapeutic skills: to be an effective problem solver in mental health practice, you need to ensure that you are creative, that you can listen, that you are able to communicate well, both verbally and non-verbally, that you can reflect, and that you are able to facilitate the service users and carers you work with to find their own solutions rather than merely instruct them.

Activities

Activity 1: reflection on a past problem

Think about a problem you have personally encountered in the past. It is best if you can think of a problem that has had an *emotional* impact on you – perhaps you have been in debt, or have been bullied, or perhaps a long-term relationship has ended.

How was the problem solved (if indeed it was)? If it was solved successfully, can you map the way in which you did it on to the stages listed above of assessment, formulation, implementation, and reflection or reassessment? If you didn't manage to solve the problem, do you think using a framework like the one described above might have helped you?

Activity 2: when the solution doesn't work

Jo, a mental health nurse, is working with Tina, a teenage girl with an eating disorder that her GP describes as 'moderate, but which may require hospitalisation in the future'. Jo visits Tina at home to carry out a routine, comprehensive assessment. Her mother is not present at the assessment (she is out at work), although her father is there. However, he does not really contribute to the assessment, remaining relatively passive during the interview even when Jo prompts him.

In concluding the assessment, Tina agrees that her eating problems may well be connected to issues with upcoming school examinations, her self-esteem and her (as Tina puts it) 'love–hate' relationship with her mother. Tina claims her mother doesn't understand her and that the constant pressure she puts on her to achieve just makes things worse. Jo and Tina agree that some family sessions with Tina and her mother might be a good first step towards helping Tina.

When Tina and her mother attend their first meeting with Jo, Tina storms out after only ten minutes stating that she knew her mother would interfere and take over, and that she couldn't see how these sessions with her mother were going to work. Clearly, at this point a collaboratively agreed potential solution hasn't worked.

What do you think Jo should do next?

When thinking about your responses, you might want to consider:

- use of the nursing process as a framework for problem solving
- the type of assessment that was carried out
- the skills of reflective practice
- who is the service user – Tina or both Tina and her family?
- whether it is too early to deem the solution a failure
- the role that clinical supervision might play (see Chapter 2).

Suggested reading

On formulation:

Johnstone, L. and Dallos, R. (eds) (2014) *Formulation in Psychology and Psychotherapy: Making Sense of People's Problems*, 2nd edn. Hove, East Sussex: Routledge.

On the specific knowledge, personal qualities and interpersonal skills needed to underpin effective problem solving in mental health:

Callaghan, P., Playle, J. and Cooper, L. (eds) (2009) *Mental Health Nursing Skills*. Oxford: Oxford University Press.

Pryjmachuk, S. (2011) The capable mental health nurse, in Pryjmachuk, S. (ed.) *Mental Health Nursing: An Evidence-based Introduction*. London: Sage.

A self-help resource for problem solving:

Fadden, G., James, C. and Pinfold, V. (2012) *Caring for Yourself: Self-help for Families and Friends Supporting People with Mental Health Problems. Booklet 5: Problem-solving and Goal Achievement*. Rethink Mental Illness/Meriden Family Programme. Birmingham: White Halo Design. Available as a PDF from: www.rethink.org/media/529020/CFY_5_Problem_Solving_and_Goal_Achievement.pdf

References

Anderson, I.M. and Fergusson, G.M. (2013) Mechanism of action of ECT, in Waite, J. and Easton, A. (eds) *The ECT Handbook*, 3rd edn. London: Royal College of Psychiatrists.

Barker, P. and Buchanan-Barker, P. (2005) *The Tidal Model: A Guide for Mental Health Professionals*. Hove: Brunner-Routledge.

Best, M. and Neuhauser, D. (2006) Walter A. Shewart, 1924, and the Hawthorne factory. *Quality and Safety in Health Care*, 15, 142–143.

British Psychological Society Division of Clinical Psychology (2011) *Good Practice Guidelines on the Use of Psychological Formulation*. Leicester: BPS.

Buzan, T. and Buzan, B. (2009) *The Mind Map Book: Unlock Your Creativity, Boost Your Memory, Change Your Life*. Harlow: BBC Active.

Callaghan, P., Playle, J. and Cooper, L. (eds) (2009) *Mental Health Nursing Skills*. Oxford: Oxford University Press.

Carey, T.A. and Pilgrim, D. (2010) Diagnosis and formulation: what should we tell the students? *Clinical Psychology and Psychotherapy*, 17, 447–454.

De Bono, E. (1970) *Lateral Thinking: A Textbook of Creativity*. Harmondsworth: Penguin.

Doran, G.T. (1981) There's a S.M.A.R.T. way to write management's goals and objectives. *Management Review*, 70, 11, 35–36.

First, M.B., Spitzer, R.L., Gibbon, M. and Williams, J.B.W. (1996) *Structured Clinical Interview for DSM-IV Axis I Disorders, Clinician Version (SCID-CV)*. Washington, DC: American Psychiatric Press.

Firth, M.T. (1999) Conversing with service users: a generic approach to mental health needs assessment. *Practice: Social Work in Action*, 11, 2, 35–48.

Han, P.K.J., Klein, W.M.P. and Arora, N.K. (2011) Varieties of uncertainty in health care: a conceptual taxonomy. *Medical Decision Making*, 31, 828–838.

Lamont, S., Brunero, S. and Russell, R. (2010) An exploratory evaluation of an action learning set within a mental health service. *Nurse Education in Practice*, 10, 298–302.

McKenna, H. (1997) *Nursing Theories and Models*. London: Routledge.

OED Online (2013) Oxford University Press. Online at www.oed.com/view/Entry/151726 (accessed 25 February 2014).

Orem, D.E. (2001) *Nursing: Concepts of Practice*, 6th edn. St Louis, MO: Mosby.

Pólya, G. (1957) *How to Solve It*, 2nd edn. Princeton, NJ: Princeton University Press.

Pryjmachuk, S. (ed.) (2011) *Mental Health Nursing: An Evidence-Based Introduction*. London: Sage.

Rimbaud, L. (2011) *8D Structured Problem Solving: A Guide to Creating High Quality 8D Reports*, 2nd edn. Breckenridge, CO: PHRED Solutions.

Rolfe, G., Jasper, M. and Freshwater, D. (eds) (2010) *Critical Reflection in Practice: Generating Knowledge for Care*, 2nd edn. Basingstoke: Palgrave-Macmillan.

Rosen, K. and Garety, P. (2005) Predicting recovery from schizophrenia: a retrospective comparison of characteristics at onset of people with single and multiple episodes. *Schizophrenia Bulletin*, 31, 3, 735–750.

Shepherd, G., Boardman, J. and Slade, M. (2008) *Making Recovery a Reality*. London: Sainsbury Centre for Mental Health.

Whitmore, J. (2009) *Coaching for Performance: GROWing Human Potential and Purpose: The Principles and Practice of Coaching and Leadership*, 4th edn. London: Nicholas Brealey Publishing.

7

The skill of offering psychoeducation

John Hyde

Introduction

'Psychoeducation has been defined as:

> the provision of information and advice about a disorder and its treatment. It usually involves an explanatory model of the symptoms and advice on how to cope with or overcome the difficulties a person may experience. It is usually of brief duration, instigated by a healthcare professional, and supported by the use of written materials.
>
> (National Institute for Health and Clinical Excellence, 2011, p. 53)

This definition from NICE suggests what psychoeducation can be, and who it can be delivered by, without stating who it should be delivered to or how it can be delivered. This chapter looks at delivering group-based psychoeducation to people with a diagnosed mental health problem. The material is primarily based on the experience of delivering psychoeducation for people with bipolar disorder, although there are aspects of this approach that would apply just as well to people with different diagnoses.

Learning objectives

After reading this chapter, you will:

- understand the evidence for using a psychoeducation approach
- be able to create topics for a psychoeducation group
- know how to set up a group
- deliver psychoeducation in a group setting
- know how to manage and evaluate a psychoeducation group.

Theoretical background

There are two aspects to delivering psychoeducation to people with a diagnosis of a psychiatric disorder. These are: the ethical aspect of informing a person about their diagnosis, and the healthcare aspect of delivering interventions that will help them cope and reduce the risk of relapse or adverse events which may at least in part be a consequence of the person's condition.

For most people in contact with mental health services, their mental health problems will usually be defined within a medical paradigm. They will receive a diagnosis of a psychiatric illness from their GP or a psychiatrist. As with any diagnosis, the person is entitled to information from staff about what their illness is, how they will be affected by it and what treatment and care they can expect to receive. The person has a right as an autonomous individual to have this information to enable them to make the best decision for them about their care.

The complexity of mental health problems can mean that some individuals have difficulties with this approach. There may be difficulties with the person's cognitions, concentration and memory, making it difficult to understand the information. The person may not view their experiences as a product of a mental health problem and therefore see the health workers' viewpoint as being at odds with their own worldview. There is a variation in how people tend to cope with information that could impact on their own sense of themselves. There are different coping styles people may use, such as 'sealing over' or using avoidance as a way of coping, or using 'integration' to try to assimilate information about a set of problems within an individual's worldview (Tait, Birchwood and Trower, 2004).

Although these tensions can present some difficulties, this does not automatically mean that the person cannot benefit from psychoeducation. The delivery of the intervention can be adapted to take into account individual difficulties. We can accept and find common ground when people have differing viewpoints. The sealing over/integration coping style can vary over individuals with time, and reflect the nature of the information they are taking on board. To begin thinking in this way, consider Mike and his experiences as introduced in Box 7.1.

Box 7.1 Introducing Mike

Mike is a 48-year-old man with a diagnosis of schizo-affective disorder. He has a long-standing belief that aliens are communicating with him, and that he has been specially chosen by them as the prophet, to pass on their message. He has had several admissions to hospital, often being detained under the Mental Health Act, after preaching in the streets his message and walking on the road stopping cars. He is prescribed depot anti-psychotic medication. He is aware that it helps to block out the communication he receives from aliens, but finds that it leaves him sedated. He accepts visits from his CPN and attends outpatient appointments at the CMHT, however he does not accept that he has a mental illness. He often asks for his medication to be reduced.

- To what extent could Mike's cognitions be impaired?
- What is Mike's understanding of his problems?
- How might a nurse work collaboratively with Mike?

The value of psychoeducation has been established for a variety of mental health diagnoses, including bipolar disorder (Colom *et al.*, 2003), schizophrenia (Xia, Merinder Lars and Belgamwar Madhvi, 2011), depression (Donker *et al.*, 2009; Tursi *et al.*, 2013), personality disorder (Wright and Jones, 2012), eating disorders (Balestrieri *et al.*, 2013) and substance misuse. In the UK the National Institute for Health and Care Excellence (NICE), recommends psychoeducation as a component of all treatments for mental health problems. In all cases, mental health problems can present in a variety of ways in terms of their symptoms, severity and presentation. This may mean using differing approaches for different people with different conditions. A brief intervention addressing the symptoms and treatment of depression may be sufficient for some people. A structured programme of psychoeducation for people with a fluctuating mental health problem may be the best approach for others (Colom, 2011). For some, like Mike introduced above, there may be ongoing issues that need to be addressed during the process.

Psychoeducation as evidence-based practice

Psychoeducation covers a wide range of approaches such as individual, family, group and family group education. It can be a stand-alone intervention or delivered as part of another therapeutic approach, such as family intervention or cognitive behavioural therapy. This chapter focuses on group psychoeducation, which offers some distinct advantages over individual approaches even though not every person is comfortable in a group-based programme (further discussion of group work can be found in Chapter 15). Advantages include, first, that delivering a programme to groups may be less resource intensive and, second, using a group-based approach may actually be more effective (Colom *et al.*, 2003).

Although psychoeducation has been in use in some form for as long as mental health care has been practised, it is only in recent years that there has been a focus on providing structured programmes. In a Cochrane review of psychoeducation for schizophrenia, effectiveness was demonstrated in medication compliance, knowledge about illness, and better social and global functioning (Xia *et al.*, 2011). However, the analysis looked at accumulated results of a variety of psychoeducational approaches of differing duration including family psychoeducation and group psychoeducation. The review team was unable to make recommendations on the duration of psychoeducation, and did not analyse group-based psychoeducation as an intervention in its own right (Xia *et al.*, 2011). Family psychoeducation may be a useful approach in reducing stress within the household and increasing coping within the family intervention approach (Fadden and Heelis, 2011). This is discussed in detail in Chapter 16.

Donker *et al.* (2009) discussed psychoeducation for depression. In this meta-analysis a variety of methods were looked at, ranging from passive strategies such as providing information leaflets to internet-based interventions and structured programmes. The overall effect demonstrated that all of these activities were effective in symptom and distress reduction. This would suggest that a stepped approach to PE might be useful depending on the nature and severity of the person's problems and the personal preference of the recipient.

A structured programme may be the most effective option for people with more severe mental health problems. The programme devised in Spain for bipolar spectrum disorders using a structured course has been shown to be beneficial in reducing symptom severity and relapse rates, with enduring benefits (Colom *et al.*, 2009). Although this 21-week programme may be difficult to implement in clinical practice, shorter programmes have also demonstrated effectiveness (Aubry *et al.*, 2012, Hoberg *et al.*, 2013).

Therapeutic approach

The following approach is derived from the psychoeducation programme for bipolar affective disorder developed by Colom, Vieta and Scott (2006). Further information about the approach is available from the National Centre for Mental Health (2014). Themes from this approach can be applied in psychoeducation for other mental health conditions. Before discussing what psychoeducation groups should be, it is important to be clear about what they are *not*. Psychoeducation is not group therapy. The purpose is to educate people about what their condition is and how to manage it. For people considering taking part in a programme it may come as a relief that members of the group are not required to discuss any personal information if they do not wish to. In fact, prior to commencing the group it may be necessary to discourage members from disclosing highly personal information. This is to prevent the person revealing information that they may later come to regret, and to avoid other members having difficulties dealing with others' personal information. Such matters may be discussed in private with the group facilitators, or the person may be encouraged to discuss with trusted people such as health and social care workers or voluntary organisations.

However, as the group progresses, often members can become closer and supportive relationships can develop, to the extent that a person does wish to disclose to the group significant traumatic events. The facilitator will need to handle these situations carefully, where it is important to try to get back on to the relevant subject matter of the day rather than be drawn into individual personal issues. This needs to be done without making the person feel uncomfortable about bringing the subject up. The facilitator will also need to be aware of the impact on other group members, and perhaps deal with them on an individual basis at the earliest opportunity.

Setting up a group

Advance preparation is key to setting up a group, and important things to consider from the outset are:

- devising the programme
- recruiting staff/acquiring skills
- involving other agencies
- awareness building
- recruitment of participants
- screening participants
- arranging a venue.

Devising the programme

Box 7.2 lists the topic areas used for bipolar disorder. Many of these can be applied to groups involving people with other mental health problems. There may also be additional topics to consider, depending on the service user group, such as hearing voices, dealing with unusual thoughts, dealing with suicidal thoughts, managing stress, stigma and discrimination, recovery, employment rights and benefits.

Box 7.2 Devising a programme

1. Introduction
2. What is bipolar disorder?
3. What causes bipolar disorder?
4. The use of medication in bipolar disorder
5. Psychological approaches
6. Lifestyle issues
7. Mood monitoring and identifying triggers
8. Early warning signs
9. Friends and families
10. Bringing it all together

Source: Bipolar Education Programme – Cymru (National Centre for Mental Health, 2014)

At this stage you should consider how to run the sessions – something that may depend on the service user group and the clinical area. Mostly, psychoeducation programmes are run with people whose mental state is currently stable, as this may well be when people are most receptive to the interventions (Colom *et al.*, 2006). However, it may still be possible to provide an intervention when people are acutely unwell, although this may need to be done with smaller groups and smaller sessions, and with careful consideration given to the impact of the sessions on the person.

Depending on the service user group you will need to decide on whether to run a closed or open group. An open group may be more applicable to an inpatient or day unit setting, due to the turnover of service users, and the familiarity with one another that may have built up outside the group setting.

Otherwise it would be better to consider a closed group, where no new members are allowed for the duration of the course. There may also be the opportunity to use a combination where participants complete an initial closed group and then can attend an additional open group for ongoing support and guidance. This is the format followed by the Life Goals Programme for bipolar disorder (Bauer and McBride, 2003). Alternatively, participants can be encouraged to attend for ongoing support through voluntary agencies such as MIND, Bipolar UK, Rethink or Hafal, if such facilities are available in the local area.

Having decided on the topics, the course will then need to be devised, alternatively using material from a structured programme such as Colom *et al.*'s (2006), Bauer and McBride's (2003) or the Bipolar Education Programme – Cymru (Craddock, Jones and Smith, 2014). The material you can use may also be dependent on the facilities and equipment available to you.

The suggested structure for a group session is as follows.

1. **Review of previous session and opportunity to discuss the session.** If any tasks were set for the participants, this would be the opportunity to discuss them among the group.

2. **Presentation of the session's topic.** This may include using slides, video clips or written material for discussion. There are resources available online, however you will need to ensure that such resources are free to use or that you have the authors' or publishers' permission to use the material.

3. **Group task or exercise.** These may be completed individually or in small groups. Possible exercises might include:

    a. drawing a life chart of your illness, as a graph, and including possible precipitants for episodes of illness

    b. causes of illness – a group sorting task using cards with possible causes and precipitants of illness or episodes of illness; the group sort these into order of importance

    c. lifestyle factors – as above, the group may sort a list of factors that can make their illness worse, and place them in order of importance

    d.   early warning signs – individually using cards, or selecting from a list of possible early warning signs

    e.   drawing up a daily mood chart or record of unusual thoughts; completing a chart for the previous week

    f.   completing an 'attitudes to medication' questionnaire for discussion

    g.   in a small group or individually, writing down the characteristics of people that have been helpful and unhelpful to you in managing your illness

    h.   devising an 'early warning signs' card that can be given to family/close friends.

The completion of each of the above tasks can be followed by participants presenting their answers and considering the issues raised.

The above are suggested exercises and you may have ideas of your own about what to do in the session. Some participants may like to share with other group members their own answers, such as showing their life chart. However, it should be made clear that doing so is voluntary as there may be personal aspects some individuals would not want to share.

4.   **Taking a break.** The timing of this may vary, and you may choose to take a break in between completing the task and participants feeding back to the group. If possible, it might be helpful to have refreshments at this stage.

5.   **Final discussion.** To finish off the session, you can begin a discussion about the topic of the day. It may be useful to have some prepared questions to begin the discussion. At this stage, participants will often engage in a discussion among themselves and the facilitator's role will be to ensure the discussion remains on topic, and that anyone who wishes to participate gets the chance and maintains a collaborative approach.

6.   **Summarise the session** and, if applicable, set any tasks to be completed for the next session. Tasks can be based on the activities completed during the session, and could be developed in greater detail (such as completing a list of early warning signs or developing a crisis plan).

As may be apparent from the above, devising the programme can be a time-intensive activity. Each session may take from 90 minutes to two hours (Colom *et al.*, 2006). In addition to the time allocated for the session, you will need time to set out the room, and allow time after it has ended to review and reflect. You may also need to allow time at the end for individual discussions with participants regarding any personal issues that have arisen that they may want to discuss. It may also be advisable to arrange supervision with other experienced practitioners to assist in review and reflection on the programme.

Who should run the group?

Psychoeducation groups have been run successfully by different professionals, including nurses (Aubry *et al.*, 2012), medical staff (de Barros Pellegrinelli *et al.*, 2013), psychologists (Candini *et al.*, 2013), occupational therapists (Eaton, 2002) and social workers (Walsh, 2010). Initial experience of the facilitation of groups and teaching can be helpful in running the group. For those less skilled, observation and an increasing level of participation can be helpful, as well as attending training events. It is advisable to have at least two people running the group. By each taking turns in leading a task, interest can be maintained. The other facilitator may be able to observe the group, deal with any individual issues and make additional comments. Although two people may run the group, it may also be useful to employ guest speakers for particular topics. For example, speakers from voluntary agencies may attend to talk about the services and support they can offer, or medical and pharmacy staff may attend to discuss medication.

Service user involvement

Some programmes of psychoeducation, such as the Self-Management Programme (Bipolar UK, 2014), are run entirely by service users, in this case by those who have experienced bipolar disorder. The experience of having mental health problems adds credibility to the teaching material if the facilitator has made use of this in their own life and can vouch for its usefulness from personal experience. It may therefore be extremely useful to have someone with experience co-facilitate, or contribute to, some sessions.

Bearing this in mind, group participants may also ask facilitators if they have experienced mental health problems in their own lives. This is a matter of personal judgement about how much to reveal if you have had some personal experience. Some degree of disclosure may help reassure participants that you understand their concerns if you have some personal experience.

Recruitment of participants

Although the efficacy of psychoeducation is well established (Rummel-Kluge, Kluge and Kissling, 2013), recruiting people for a group can be a time-intensive process. One can advertise with posters in health care settings, and with emails to health professionals and agencies working with service users. However, these ways of recruiting can often be overlooked or ignored. Speaking directly to agencies such as community mental health teams and giving out leaflets to pass on to service users can stimulate interest. It is helpful therefore to know in advance that you have sufficient people wanting to attend, before organising the actual event.

Prior to accepting people onto a programme, it would be advisable to contact all participants for the group to ensure that they will be able to benefit.

Some questions to consider are as follows.

1.   What are your expectations about the course?

This is to check whether the course will meet the person's expectations and needs.

2.   Do you have a diagnosis from a psychiatrist for the condition that the group addresses?

This may be less relevant for groups that are not condition specific. However, a person with a diagnosis of depression will gain very limited benefit and may not feel part of a group specifically for people with bipolar disorder.

3.   Do you mind if we speak to a professional involved in your care?

Often attendance is at the suggestion of a person involved. It can help to check if they think the person will benefit, or if they have any concerns about the person's participation.

4.   Do you have any other diagnosed mental health problems?

This will not automatically mean that the person should not participate, however if their primary diagnosis differs from the group's main subject matter the person may not benefit from attending.

5.   Do you have any current issues with drugs or alcohol?

If the person has ongoing problems, and is likely to attend while under the influence of drugs or alcohol, this can be disruptive and they may not benefit from participation.

6.   When and where would you prefer to attend the group?

This is to get an idea of when to run the group: during the day or evening.

Having compiled a list of participants, facilitators will be aware of how many groups they will need to plan for, also being aware that more people may make contact with the intention of taking part, which may mean placing them on a waiting list and informing them of the likely commencement date of the next group.

Organising the group

Group numbers should be around 15 to start with and preferably no fewer than 10. Anticipate that up to one-third of participants will drop out of the course. This may be due to them feeling that they do not want to take part, but also because participants often drop out due to other issues, including ill-health, family matters, difficulty getting to the venue and so on.

Ideally the venue should be a room with sufficient space for the members, with access to a projector and screen if you are using a computer. The seating can be arranged in a circle, or around a table in the style of a conference meeting. The latter allows for communication between members, the ability to take notes easily and is more formal than sitting in a circle; this makes it more in tune with an educational intervention. It is important to pay attention to the layout and seating, to achieve the right balance to facilitate discussion.

Group members ideally should have access to refreshments – water, tea, coffee, biscuits – as well as writing materials to use during group tasks. Booking the venue itself can sometimes be an issue, due to financial and other issues. Ideally, the group should be held away from local mental health service premises, as this is more conducive to the participatory and educational aspect of the programme. Venues that may be available at no, or minimal, cost include community centres, local educational institutions, church halls and general hospital premises. The venue should also be easily accessible for group members, by public transport or car.

Running the group

The first session

The following is an outline example of the first session of a psychoeducation group. This will lay the foundation for the following groups and set the scene for how following groups will be run.

1. Introduction
Facilitators will introduce themselves, giving some professional background information where applicable. Name badges will be given out, so that everyone knows one another's names. Housekeeping matters will be addressed: location of fire exits and lavatories, refreshments, etc.

2. Rules of the group
There are some rules that you may have in mind for the group, but it is also helpful to ask participants what rules they think should apply. Examples include:

a.   respect one another

b.   allow one another time to talk

c.   turn up on time

d.   attend regularly

e.   maintain the group's confidentiality

f.   take an active part in the discussion.

3. Warm-up exercise

This may be some exercise to help the group members get to know one another. There are different types of 'icebreaker' you can use, depending on your preference. One example is getting people into pairs and then getting them to ask each other some questions (see Box 7.3). Then each person feeds back to the group what they have learned about the other person.

Box 7.3 Getting to know you

1. What is your neighbour's name?
2. Where do they come from?
3. What is their favourite TV programme?
4. What is their favourite holiday destination?
5. What is their favourite drink?

This might address why psychoeducation is helpful, and what will be covered over this course. It may consider how people can get the most out of the programme, and how sessions will be structured, giving examples from following sessions.

Participants should be encouraged to ask questions and make comments during the presentation. However, if any points raised are going to create a long discussion, it is useful to suggest that the group return to this topic during the discussion period after the break.

4. Break

5. Discussion

This is an opportunity for the group to ask questions and discuss their own aims about what they hope to gain from taking part. This also allows the opportunity to discuss any earlier points raised in greater detail. If the previous steps have created an atmosphere where participants feel comfortable with one another, then the discussion will be more successful and require less prompting from the facilitators.

Conclusion

The effective running of a psychoeducation group requires prior planning to develop resources, recruit staff to run the group and participants to take part in the group, as well as consideration of the setting and logistics of running a group.

The above model of psychoeducation is based on an established and well-researched programme (Colom, 2011) and can form a template to use this approach with a wide range of mental health problems.

Activities

Activity 1

In setting up a psychoeducation group in your local area, who could you involve in the programme and what might they contribute? Consider:

- service users
- health and social care professionals
- voluntary-sector organisations
- carers/relatives.

Activity 2

What further skills and support might you need to set up a programme? Consider:

- training
- supervision
- managerial/organisational support.

Key points

1. Psychoeducation is an effective way of helping people manage their illness.
2. Psychoeducation can be used with many different mental health problems.
3. Planning is essential for a successful group.
4. It is not group therapy.
5. Choose and set up your venue with care.
6. Discussion between group participants is necessary for a successful group.
7. The facilitator's role is to guide the discussion and keep the group safe more than it is about teaching.
8. Group participants have their own knowledge and expertise about their illness, make use of these assets.

Suggested reading

Colom, F., Vieta, E. and Scott, J. (2006) *Psychoeducation Manual for Bipolar Disorder.* New York: Cambridge University Press.

A psychoeducation manual and description of a 21-week programme for bipolar disorder. This has formed the basis for research into psychoeducation.

Bauer, M.S. and McBride, L.M. (2003) *Structured Group Psychotherapy for Bipolar Disorder: The Life Goals Program*, 2nd edn. New York: Springer Publishing Company.

Although this book is getting old now, the programme described is still in use throughout the world.

References

Aubry, J.M., Charmillot, A., Aillon, N., Bourgeois, P., Mertel, S., Nerfin, F., Romailler, G., Stauffer, M.J., Gex-Fabry, M. and De Andres, R.D. (2012) Long-term impact of the life goals group therapy program for bipolar patients. *Journal of Affective Disorders*, 136, 889–894.

Balestrieri, M., Isola, M., Baiano, M. and Ciano, R. (2013) Psychoeducation in binge eating disorder and EDNOS: a pilot study on the efficacy of a 10-week and a 1-year continuation treatment. *Eating and Weight Disorders*, 18, 45–51.

Bauer, M.S. and McBride, L.M. (2003) *Structured Group Psychotherapy for Bipolar Disorder: The Life Goals Program*, 2nd edn. New York: Springer Publishing Company.

Bipolar UK (2014) Self management. Online at www.bipolaruk.org.uk/self-management/ (accessed 6 June 2014).

Candini, V., Buizza, C., De Girolamo, G., Ferrari, C., Caldera, M.T., Nobili, G., Pioli, R., Sacchetti, E., Saviotti, F.M., Seggioli, G. and Zanini, A. (2013) A study of effectiveness of structured group psychoeducation for bipolar patients. A controlled trial in Italy. *European Psychiatry*, 28, Suppl. 1.

Colom, F. (2011) Keeping therapies simple: psychoeducation in the prevention of relapse in affective disorders. *British Journal of Psychiatry*, 198, 338–340.

Colom, F., Vieta, E. and Scott, J. (2006) *Psychoeducation Manual for Bipolar Disorder*. New York: Cambridge University Press.

Colom, F., Vieta, E., Martinez-Aran, A., Reinares, M., Goikolea, J.M., Benabarre, A., Torrent, C., Comes, M., Corbella, B., Parramon, G. and Corominas, J. (2003) A randomized trial on the efficacy of group psychoeducation in the prophylaxis of recurrences in bipolar patients whose disease is in remission. *Archives of General Psychiatry*, 60, 402–407.

Colom, F., Vieta, E., Sanchez-Moreno, J., Palomino-Otiniano, R., Reinares, M., Goikolea, J.M., Benabarre, A. and Martinez-Aran, A. (2009) Group psychoeducation for stabilised bipolar disorders: 5-year outcome of a randomised clinical trial. *British Journal of Psychiatry*, 194, 260–265.

Craddock, N., Jones, I. and Smith, D. (2014) *Bipolar Education Programme – Cymru*. Online at http://ncmh.info/bepcymru/ (accessed 6 June 2014).

De Barros Pellegrinelli, K., de O Costa, L.F., Silval, K.I., Dias, V.V., Roso, M.C., Bandeira, M., Colom, F. and Moreno, R.A. (2013) Efficacy of psychoeducation on symptomatic and functional recovery in bipolar disorder. *Acta Psychiatrica Scandinavica*, 127, 153–158.

Donker, T., Griffiths, K.M., Cuijpers, P. and Christensen, H. (2009) Psychoeducation for depression, anxiety and psychological distress: a meta-analysis. *BMC Medicine*, 7, 79.

Eaton, P. (2002) Psychoeducation in acute mental health settings: is there a role for occupational therapists? *British Journal of Occupational Therapy*, 65, 321–326.

Fadden, G. and Heelis, R. (2011) The Meriden Family Programme: lessons learned over 10 years. *Journal of Mental Health*, 20, 79–88.

Hoberg, A.A., Ponto, J., Nelson, P.J. and Frye, M.A. (2013) Group interpersonal and social rhythm therapy for bipolar depression. *Perspectives in Psychiatric Care*, 49, 226–234.

National Centre for Mental Health (2014) *Bipolar Education Programme Cymru*. Cardiff: National Centre For Mental Health. Online at http://ncmh.info/bepcymru/ (accessed 4 December 2015).

National Institute for Health and Clinical Excellence (2011) Common mental health disorders: identification and pathways to care. *Clinical Guideline* 123. London: National

Institute for Health and Clinical Excellence. Online at www.nice.org.uk (accessed 4 December 2015).

Rummel-Kluge, C., Kluge, M. and Kissling, W. (2013) Frequency and relevance of psycho-education in psychiatric diagnoses: results of two surveys five years apart in German-speaking European countries. *BMC Psychiatry*, 13, 170.

Tait, L., Birchwood, M. and Trower, P. (2004) Adapting to the challenge of psychosis: personal resilience and the use of sealing-over (avoidant) coping strategies. *British Journal of Psychiatry*, 185, 410–415.

Tursi, M.F., Baes, C., Camacho, F.R., Tofoli, S.M. and Juruena, M.F. (2013) Effectiveness of psychoeducation for depression: a systematic review. *Australian and New Zealand Journal of Psychiatry*, 47, 1019–1031.

Walsh, J.F. (2010) *Psychoeducation in Mental Health*. Chicago, IL: Lyceum Books, Inc.

Wright, K. and Jones, F. (2012) Therapeutic alliances in people with borderline personality disorder. *Mental Health Practice*, 16, 31–35.

Xia, J., Merinder Lars, B. and Belgamwar Madhvi, R. (2011) Psychoeducation for schizophrenia. *Cochrane Database of Systematic Reviews*. Online at www.mrw.interscience.wiley.com/cochrane/clsysrev/articles/CD002831/frame.html (accessed 4 December 2015).

8

Skills to challenge unhelpful thoughts

Jo Sullivan

Introduction

In this chapter I introduce some of the techniques that are used to help service users identify, challenge or reframe unhelpful thoughts associated with their problems. These techniques are the basic components of cognitive behavioural therapy (CBT).

The main aim of any therapeutic intervention is to relieve suffering and distress. Poorly defined or delivered therapeutic interventions may be harmful to the service user. It is therefore essential that any therapeutic intervention forms part of a coherent treatment plan, and that the practitioner has the relevant skills and supervision to safely undertake the work.

Experiencing unpleasant or distressing thoughts is a natural response to specific painful events or experiences, such as loss or bereavement. CBT is concerned with thoughts that are persistently negative, unhelpful and distressing, of a type that are maintained by distorted, biased and restricted thinking patterns. This chapter will explore the practical application of the following cognitive behavioural techniques:

- thought records or diaries
- Socratic dialogue or guided discovery
- behavioural experiments.

These approaches have the overarching aim of monitoring symptoms, along with identifying and addressing unhelpful triggers and patterns of thoughts, emotions and behaviour. The introduction of new ideas or alternative information is intended to help the service user develop a more balanced and helpful thinking style.

Learning objectives

After reading this chapter, you will:

- understand the basic theory behind the cognitive behavioural approach
- identify self-defeating thoughts that cognitive behavioural techniques aim to address
- describe specific cognitive behavioural interventions that help service users to monitor, challenge and reframe unhelpful thoughts
- know how to work collaboratively with service users to help them identify and change unhelpful thinking patterns.

A brief history of CBT, and the rationale for identifying and challenging negative thoughts

Behaviour therapy emerged in the late 1800s and was based on the principles of animal learning. Pavlov (1927) and Skinner (1953) investigated classical and operant conditioning, which are the relationships between external stimuli and behaviour. This led to the development of treatment approaches for a range of psychological problems including anxiety disorders and depression based on changing external conditions to bring about change in behaviour.

Behaviour therapy was not concerned with cognitions (internal mental processes such as thoughts), as these could not be observed directly. However, people use language and thoughts to make sense of what is happening to and around them. Treatment failures using behavioural therapy alone and the observation that people tend to generate their own explanations for things led to an interest in cognitions.

In 1975 Meichenbaum developed a cognitive approach which demonstrated that changing thoughts led to changes in behaviour. Later, Beck and colleagues (1979) showed that changing negative thinking in depression could assist recovery. He suggested that negative thoughts originate in attitudes and beliefs formed in childhood. These beliefs are triggered by experiences in the 'here and now', which maintain the negative cycle of distress. Beck *et al.* (1979) introduced the cognitive triad, which include beliefs that the individual holds about themselves, others and the world. For example, an individual may believe 'I am worthless, others are superior and the world is unsafe.' The interplay between these beliefs reinforces negative thinking.

Beck and colleagues (1979) then developed cognitive behaviour therapy (CBT) for depression. This remains one of the most widely applied and evaluated psychological therapy approaches. Central to CBT is the impact of negative thoughts on the development and maintenance of depression. Identifying and challenging or reframing negative thinking has become a cornerstone of the cognitive behavioural approach.

Randomised controlled trails and meta-analyses show that CBT is an effective intervention in the treatment of depression, panic disorder, generalised anxiety and obsessive compulsive disorder (DoH, 2001). CBT is a problem-focused psychosocial intervention based on the principles of collaboration, detailed assessment, psychoeducation, testing out theories and learning new skills. A formulation of the service user's problem leads to clear treatment goals (Westbrook and Kirk, 2007).

Thinking about thinking

CBT defines different levels of thinking. Beck *et al.* (1979) identified three levels of cognitions: negative automatic thoughts, dysfunctional assumptions and core beliefs.

Negative automatic thoughts (NATs)

NATs are 'surface level' cognitions. They appear to 'pop' into one's mind in an involuntary manner. NATs are accepted as fact even if they are not always supported by the things the individual knows to be true. They are maintained by thinking errors, which are biased, restricted and emotionally laden. They are amenable to change but often form part of a vicious circle that maintains the problem (Simmons and Griffiths, 2009).

Dysfunctional assumptions

These are the rules the individual lives by, often expressed as 'should' or 'if ... then' statements. Dysfunctional assumptions bridge the gap between NATs and core beliefs. They are not always accessible to the individual because they are taken for granted. They are rigid, over-generalised and extreme. They do not reflect normal human experience and they can prevent rather than facilitate goals. Breaking life 'rules' can lead to extreme and excessive distress (Hawton *et al.*, 1989).

Core beliefs

Core beliefs are the very essence of how an individual views themselves, others, the world and the future. They shape our identity. Core beliefs develop over time, and are influenced by life circumstances and experiences. They are rigid, inflexible and resistant to change. They are maintained by the individual's tendency to attend only to information that supports the core belief.

Thinking errors

Beck (1967) identified several common thinking errors that shape and maintain unhelpful thinking patterns. These are described in Tables 8.1 to 8.4.

Table 8.1 Extreme thinking errors

Thinking error	Descriptor
All-or-nothing thinking	Black-and-white thinking: if it isn't perfect then it's a total failure
Catastrophising	Thinking the very worst thing will happen – for example, 'I'm not having a panic attack, I'm having a heart attack'

Table 8.2 Selective thinking errors

Thinking error	Descriptor
Over-generalisation	Everything is viewed as negative; the positives are ignored
Mental filter	Focusing on a single negative detail
Magnification or minimisation	Exaggerating the importance of own problem; failure to consider context
Discounting positives	Here the focus is on negative attributes – small things become exaggerated and distorted; words such as 'never', 'always' or 'every' may be clues to the presence of selective attention

Table 8.3 Intuition thinking errors

Thinking error	Descriptor
Mind reading	Making assumptions about other people's motives or predicting the worst without evidence
Fortune telling	Anticipating that things will end in a negative manner
Emotional reasoning	Assuming that one's own negative emotions reflect the truth

Table 8.4 Self-reproach thinking errors

Thinking error	Descriptor
Rigid rules	Engaging in a set of fixed ideas about how self and others should behave; exaggerating negative consequences if rules are not adhered to
Unfair judgements	Holding self personally responsible for events beyond one's control
Name calling	Placing extremely negative and emotionally laden labels on oneself or others, such as 'I'm a useless piece of rubbish'

Box 8.1 summarises key points covered in this chapter so far.

Box 8.1 CBT key points

- CBT is a psychosocial intervention that focuses on the interplay between thoughts, feelings, emotions and behaviour, and the vicious circle that maintains problems.
- It is widely applied and evaluated, and has been shown to be effective in the treatment of various psychological problems including depression and anxiety disorders.
- The influence of unhelpful thoughts in the development and maintenance of problems is recognised and understood. Helping service users to change their thinking style reduces distress.
- Beck (1967) introduced the role of thinking errors in reinforcing the individual's negative beliefs about themselves, others, the world and the future.

Cognitive behavioural techniques in clinical practice

Changing unhelpful thinking

Cognitive restructuring is the process of replacing unhelpful thoughts with thoughts that are more accurate and useful. This involves two basic steps:

1. identify the thinking errors or beliefs that influence the distressing emotion

2. evaluate them for their accuracy and usefulness using logic and evidence, modifying or replacing the thoughts with others that are more balanced.

Padesky and Greenberger (1995) offer a cognitive therapy skills checklist that identifies automatic thoughts, and suggest experiments to test these. They also offer methods to identify core beliefs and assumptions, recognising the connection between thoughts and moods.

There are three basic techniques that facilitate restructuring of surface level cognitions:

1. thought records help to identify unhelpful thoughts and encourage the service user to begin the process of challenging thinking biases or distortions

2. Socratic questioning and 'down arrow' techniques gather more detailed information about the problem and introduce uncertainty about the conviction in which a thought is held

3. finally, behavioural experiments test out the accuracy of thoughts and help the service user to form a more balanced and helpful belief.

Thought records or diaries

Thought records are relatively straightforward to use. They can be practised in session and as a homework task. They help the service user to gather detailed information about their problem.

Thought records allow the service user to recognise and label thoughts and feelings, and to identify patterns and triggers. Often service users are unaware of or are unable to recognise emotions. Psychologist and researcher Robert Plutchnick has studied emotions extensively. He has identified and paired eight primary emotions; these are Joy vs Sadness, Trust vs Disgust, Fear vs Anger and Surprise vs Anticipation (see Plutchnick (1980) for more detailed understanding of emotional recognition and meaning).

Completed thought records demonstrate changes in thoughts, feelings and behaviour over time. This helps to build up a picture of the service user's problem and also provides evidence for positive changes. Some excellent thought records or diaries exist (Beck *et al.*, 1979; Padesky and Greenberger, 1995; Westbrook and Kirk, 2007); an example is given in Table 8.5.

Table 8.5 An example of a thought record

Rating scale 0–10 (0 = no distress, 5 = moderately distressed, 10 = extremely distressed)

Date and time	Event or behaviour	Feeling	Thought and rating of distress	Evidence to support NAT	Evidence against NAT	Re-rate level of distress
20.02.14 15.00 hrs	Failed driv-ing test	Angry, upset	I can't do anything right. I always fail everything. Level of distress: 10	I've failed my GCSEs and I didn't get the Saturday job.	I re-sat exams and passed. I've been offered a place at uni. Most people fail driving exam the first time.	Level of distress: 4

There are several steps to completing a thought record. The service user is helped to identify the following:

• the event or behaviour that precedes unpleasant emotions

Consider prompts such as 'What was occurring? What were you doing immediately prior to the strong feeling? Where were you? Who else was present? What time of day or day of the week was it?'

• label the unpleasant emotion and rate distress

Include psychoeducation about primary emotions and their meaning.

- recognise thinking error or NATs

A worksheet of common thinking errors can be an effective prompt. Information gathered during the assessment and formulation phase of work will provide some clues about the likely NATs.

- review evidence for and against the belief

Encourage the service user to work systematically through the evidence that supports and contradicts the thinking error or NAT. It takes practice to focus on both positives and negatives.

- re-rate level of distress

Re-rating distress levels shows changes in the individual's thoughts and feelings. It demonstrates the success of the technique, enhancing confidence and encouraging future use.

In the example in Table 8.5 the individual is engaging in several thinking errors, including all-or-nothing thinking, over-generalising, discounting positives, and emotional reasoning. In order to further develop insight, the thought record could be enhanced over time so that the individual begins to name the thinking errors and directly challenge them. This example demonstrates that, simply by exploring the evidence for and against the belief, the individual is able to significantly reduce their level of distress.

Socratic questions and guided discovery

Socratic questions, or guided discovery, assist an individual to reframe unhelpful thoughts during the therapeutic conversation. These techniques build on the collaborative nature and the spirit of curiosity in the CBT approach. While the terms are often used interchangeably, there are some differences in approach.

Guided discovery is based on asking questions that allow information to be brought into the individual's awareness. It prompts the individual to recognise and evaluate their unquestioned beliefs. Guided discovery uses questions such as:

- What's the evidence?
- What alternative views are there?
- What is the effect of thinking the way you do?
- What thinking errors are you making when you come to that conclusion? (Burns, 1980)

Socratic questions are at the heart of critical thinking. This is the process we use to reflect on, access and judge the assumptions underlying our own and others' ideas and behaviour. Padesky and Greenberger (1995) suggest that there are four main types of question that make up the Socratic process, as follows.

Clarification:

- What exactly does this mean?
- Can you give me an example?
- What's the worst thing that can happen?

Probing assumptions:

- What else could we assume if that were true?
- What would happen if that were correct/incorrect?

Probing rationale, reasons and evidence:

- Why is that happening?
- How do you know this is true?
- What's the evidence for and against this?

Probing implications and consequences:

- If X happens, then what?
- Why is X important?
- Is there a more helpful way to view the situation?

An example of Socratic dialogue is given in Box 8.2.

Box 8.2 Socratic dialogue in action

Kim is crying because she believes that Jack has been standing outside her door laughing at her. Kim is sensitive about her appearance and becomes preoccupied with the idea that others think that she is ugly.

> Kim: I want to make a complaint. Jack has been standing outside my door all morning, laughing at me.
> Practitioner: I can see that you are upset. I would be upset too if I thought someone had been laughing at me. What makes you think that Jack was laughing at you?

Kim: He knew that I was going to get dressed and he knows that I hate the way I look. I told him at breakfast.

Practitioner: Why might Jack think the way you look is funny?

Kim: All men think I'm funny looking. I've been called ugly all my life.

Practitioner: Is it possible that Jack was laughing at something else?

Kim: I suppose so, but I don't think so.

Practitioner: What else might he have been laughing at?

Kim: Well, he was sitting with Tony after breakfast and I know that Tony's always telling jokes.

Practitioner: So Jack could have been laughing with Tony?

Kim: Yes, I suppose so.

Practitioner: OK, so apart from you hearing Jack laughing this morning, is there anything else that makes you think that Jack may think negatively about you?

Kim: No that's why I was so upset. I thought that Jack was my friend.

Practitioner: OK, you've said that you thought Jack was laughing at you and that made you feel upset, but you've also said that it's possible that Jack was laughing with Tony. You've no other reason to believe that Jack doesn't like you in fact you've always been friends. Which of these possibilities do you think is most likely to be true?

Kim: I think that Jack was laughing at Tony not me.

Practitioner: How do you feel now?

Kim: Much better. A bit bad for thinking that about Jack. I'll go and speak to him. Thank you.

Delusional beliefs are unlikely to respond to rational debate. There is a risk that in practice clinicians feel obliged to inform the service user that their beliefs are incorrect for fear that they may reinforce the delusion. It is possible to attend to the service user's emotional distress and to promote problem-solving strategies without contradicting the individual's beliefs. Chadwick, Birchwood and Trower (1996) and Morrison *et al.* (2003), among others, have demonstrated the efficacy of cognitive behavioural approaches for individuals suffering from psychotic illnesses. In the scenario in Box 8.2 the practitioner validates Kim's feelings and encourages her to talk. Kim is not directly challenged nor is she persuaded of Jack's innocence. Kim is encouraged to consider alternative explanations, and to explore the evidence for and against her belief. Kim is able to generate an alternative perspective and consequently feels less distressed.

Problems in challenging thinking errors and NATs

The techniques to help service users identify thinking errors and NATs are relatively straightforward. It is more difficult to reframe negative thoughts because they are often triggered by strong emotions that, in the moment, prevent clear thinking. The techniques can work only if the individual believes in them. Similarly, if the practitioner assumes that the belief is justifiable it may interfere with the process. Another limitation is the length of time and amount of practice needed to support lasting change. Putting a structure around the process, generating new evidence with the service user and having them test it out, strengthens the validity of the approach (Hawton *et al.*, 1989).

Behavioural experiments

A third technique that will help individuals challenge negative thoughts is behavioural experiments. These can be targeted at the individual's thoughts, feelings or behaviour. Making a change to any one of these areas will eventually effect change in all three. In a behavioural experiment the individual makes a prediction about their belief and tests it out. This process either confirms the prediction or facilitates change.

Behavioural experiments can include active or observational experiments (Bennett-Levy, 2003). Active experiments involve the individual doing something to generate information. This may include trying new behaviours and observing the consequences. Observational experiments involve gathering information through observing events or interactions between other people. Active experiments are more challenging but are more likely to reinforce learning. Both types of behavioural experiment are more powerful than routine verbal discussions.

There are several steps to setting up a behavioural experiment, as described below.

Identify the negative automatic thought and the predicted outcome
The purpose and rationale for the experiment should become clear from the individual's thought records or through Socratic dialogue. Once the negative thought has been identified, further questions such as, 'And if that were true, what then?' will help to reveal the predicted outcome. For example, Susan believes that her boss attends only meetings that she leads. She believes he is checking up on her because he thinks she is incompetent. The practitioner asks, 'If you are incompetent what would that mean?' Susan replies, 'If I am incompetent I will lose my job.' Susan's NAT is that she is incompetent and she predicts that she will lose her job.

Rate strength of belief about NAT and predicted outcome
Rating strength of belief allows the individual to measure change before and after the experiment. This helps to evaluate the results.

Review existing evidence for and against
Reviewing the evidence that supports and contradicts the belief helps to clarify what exactly needs to be reframed. The process itself can begin to challenge the strength of conviction in the belief.

In Susan's case it is likely that this will reveal that she is over-generalising, mind reading, fortune telling and engaging in emotional reasoning.

Decide on a plan of action to test out the truth of the prediction
It is important to spend time clarifying what negative thought and prediction is being tested out. Poorly defined negative thoughts or thinking errors will lead to ineffective behavioural experiments. Spending time considering what may go wrong helps to refine the process.

Identifying a clear prediction can be difficult. It is impossible to measure an outcome such as 'it will be awful'. Clarifying questions, such as 'How would you know if the situation was awful?' or 'What would be happening to you if the situation was awful?', may be useful.

Record results
Keeping a record of results helps to strengthen any learning that has occurred. Collating outcomes from several behavioural experiments can help to identify patterns or themes.

Evaluate the conclusion
The individual should be encouraged to reflect on how they can apply any new learning and to review whether any further experiments could lead to more balanced perspectives.

Box 8.3 gives an example of a behavioural experiment.

Box 8.3 Behavioural experiments in action

Nurse: Are you planning to attend your clinical team meeting this week?
John: I don't know. Whenever I do, I leave feeling frustrated.
Nurse: Why is that?
John: I've got a lot of questions about my medication, but I don't like to ask about it.
Nurse: What do you think will happen if you do ask questions?
John: I think they'll think I'm stupid. I worry that they'll think I don't want to take the medication and they won't let me go home.
Nurse: On a scale of 0–100, 0 being not at all and 100 being completely, how much do you believe your worrying thoughts?
John: About 90 per cent.
Nurse: What's the evidence to support your worrying thoughts?
John: Well, the team know that I failed all my exams in school. I go red when I speak and I look stupid. I should already know why they picked that medication because I should know about my illness.
Nurse: Is there evidence against your beliefs?

John: Yes, if I was stupid I wouldn't have thought of the question in the first place. I don't think other people are stupid when they ask questions in the meeting. The psychologist told me that my IQ is 110 and that asking questions shows that I'm interested and want to learn about my illness. Just because I go red doesn't mean I'm stupid, just anxious. Most people would be anxious going into their team meeting.

Nurse: What can you do to test out your prediction that the team will think you are stupid and don't want to take your medication?

John: In the clinical team meeting on Tuesday, I'll ask the doctor why he has chosen that particular medication. I will see whether he answers me directly or not. I will watch the reaction of the team members. If he lets me go on leave I'll know that he trusts me to take my medication.

When John attended the meeting the team were encouraging and the doctor told him that his question was good and his concerns understandable. He took time to explain to John why he had chosen the particular medication. John felt anxious before he asked the question, but calm and pleased with himself afterwards. He was able to reframe his belief and concluded that, 'The team appeared to be impressed by my question and encouraging. The belief that the team think I am stupid is now 5 per cent.'

Table 8.6 gives an example of a behavioural experiment record.

Table 8.6 Recording behavioural experiments

Date	Target NAT	Experiment	Prediction	Results	Conclusion
	What is the negative belief that I am testing? How much do I believe this? (0–100%)	Design an experiment that will test your belief, facing a situation you would otherwise avoid or trying something new	State what you think will happen, and review the evidence for and against your prediction	Record what actually happened. What did you observe? How does it fit with your predictions?	What did I learn? What does this mean about my original belief/ assumption? How much do I believe that now? (0–100%)

Conclusion

This chapter has touched on basic principles of the cognitive behavioural approach and its relevance to specific psychological problems, including depression and anxiety. The approach focuses on the interplay between thoughts, feelings, emotions and behaviour. This chapter has explored unhelpful thoughts and their role in maintaining problems. Three specific techniques were outlined that are widely used in cognitive behavioural approaches to reframe unhelpful thoughts:

1. thought records
2. Socratic dialogue and guided discovery
3. behavioural experiments.

These techniques allow the service user to monitor symptoms, recognise and label emotions and thoughts, and to identify patterns and themes that lead to distress.

'Surface level' thoughts were described, including thinking errors and NATs that are easily accessible to the service user, commonly reported to clinicians and amenable to change. This chapter shows how these techniques can be used to help people to challenge biased, distorted or restricted thinking, freeing them up to view themselves, others, the world and the future in a more positive light.

Activities

Activity 1
To consolidate your learning it is important to review the four main ideas outlined in this chapter and to consider the implications for your practice. Working through Table 8.7, take ten minutes to describe what you have learned about each idea and how this will influence your practice.

Table 8.7 Consolidating learning

Thinking errors	Thought records
• Can you name them? • When might you use them?	• Name the steps in completing a thought record
Socratic questions and guided discovery • Can you name the type of questions asked? • What are the advantages of this approach?	**Behavioural experiments** • When might you use a behavioural experiment? • Can you name the steps involved?

Activity 2
CBT is based on the idea that psychological difficulties are an extension of normal processes. With this in mind, use a thought record to reframe one of your own unhelpful thoughts (see Table 8.8). Practising on yourself will improve your confidence in the technique before you guide a service user through the process.

Table 8.8 Reframing personal thoughts

Date and time	Event or behaviour	Feeling	Thought and rating of distress	Evidence to support NAT	Evidence against NAT	Re-rate level of distress

Activity 3
Discuss with your supervisor what you have learned from reading this chapter. Consider whether you might benefit from further training in CBT as part of your personal development plan.

Suggested reading

Padesky, C. and Greenberger, D. (1995) *Clinician's Guide to Mind over Mood*. New York: Guilford Press.

This is a well-regarded text in the field, with good worked examples of thought records and dialogue exemplars.

References

Beck, A.T. (1967) *Depression: Clinical, Experimental and Theoretical Aspects*. New York: Harper & Row.

Beck, A.T., Rush, A.J., Shaw, B.F. and Emery, G. (1979) *Cognitive Therapy of Depression*. New York: Guilford Press.

Bennett-Levy, J. (2003) Mechanisms of change in cognitive therapy: the case of automatic thought records and behavioural experiments. *Behavioural and Cognitive Psychotherapy*, 31, 261–277.

Burns, D. (1980) *Feeling Good: The New Mood Therapy*. New York: William Morrow.

Chadwick, P., Birchwood, M. and Trower, P. (1996) *Cognitive Therapy for Delusions, Voices and Paranoia*. Chichester: Wiley.

Department of Health (2001) *Treatment Choice in Psychological Therapies and Counselling*. London: Department of Health.

Hawton, K., Salkovskis, P., Kirk, J. and Clark, D. (1989) *Cognitive Behaviour Therapy for Psychiatric Problems. A Practical Guide*. Oxford: Oxford University Press.

Meichenbaum, D. (1975) Self-instructional methods, in Kanfer, F. and Goldstein, P. (eds) *Helping People Change: A Textbook of Methods* (pp. 357–391). New York: Pergamon.

Morrison, A., Renton, J., Dunn, A., Williams, S. and Bentall, R. (2003) *Cognitive Therapy for Psychosis. A Formulation Based Approach*. London: Routledge.

Padesky, C. and Greenberger, D. (1995) *Clinician's Guide to Mind over Mood*. New York: Guilford Press.

Pavlov, I. (1927) *Conditional Reflexes: An Investigation of the Physiological Activity of the Cerebral Cortex*. London: Oxford University Press.

Plutchnick, R. (1980) *Emotion: Theory, Research and Experience, Vol. 1 Theories of Emotion*. New York: Academic.

Simmons, J. and Griffiths, R. (2009) *CBT for Beginners*. London: Sage.

Skinner, B.F. (1953) *Science and Human Behaviour*. New York: Macmillan.

Westbrook, D. and Kirk, J. (2007) *An introduction to Cognitive Behaviour Therapy: Skills and Applications*. London: Sage.

q

Validation skills applied to people with dementia

Paul Bickerstaffe and Amanda King

Introduction

Before reading this chapter consider the following questions.

- What makes you the person you are?
- How do you engage and connect with other people?
- How important is it to you to be able to share your values, feelings and emotions with others?

We are all individuals, thus our answers to the above questions will vary from person to person. However, it is likely that the need to communicate with others effectively, and for other people to actively listen and understand, is a common theme throughout your answers. This will be no different from the person who has a dementia.

The aim of this chapter is to provide the reader with a range of therapeutic approaches and skills that can be used to validate a person's experiences. While it will draw upon some of the principles and skills of validation therapy, this is not a chapter on validation therapy per se.

Learning objectives

After reading this chapter, you will:

- understand the principles on which validation techniques are based
- recognise the challenges faced by people with dementia in maintaining their identity and expressing themselves
- be able to use therapeutic skills that facilitate validation.

People with dementia have needs similar to those of other people. However, the symptoms of the disease can make it difficult for others to understand what those needs are. Recently in England the Department of Health launched a new nursing vision and strategy for dementia care (DoH, 2013), inviting healthcare professionals to improve the quality of care and hence quality of life for people with dementia. The focus of this strategy is on understanding and caring for the complex needs of people with dementia, acknowledging their physical, mental health, emotional and spiritual needs within a context of thinking about the whole person, their uniqueness, their story and noticing the things that matter to them. In aspiring to meet this standard of care delivery the nurse will need to draw upon a range of therapeutic skills that will enable them to have a deeper understanding of the overall experience of dementia, including the feelings and emotions felt by the person with dementia. Box 9.1 lists some of these skills.

Box 9.1 Therapeutic skills that support a validation approach

- Validation techniques
- Positive Person Work
- Reminiscence
- Sonas (Activating the Potential to Communicate)
- The End of Life Namaste Care Program for People with Dementia

The Nursing and Midwifery Council (NMC) in its Guidance for the Care of Older People (2009) recognises that a nurse working with older people must possess the skills of empathy and compassion. Empathy is described as having a feeling for what someone is going through, putting yourself in the person's place and imagining how you might feel. The value of helpfulness, friendliness, warmth, cheerfulness, kindness and decency is also emphasised.

The principles of validation therapy

Naomi Feil developed the Validation Method for communication with people that have Alzheimer's-type dementia; it is also known as Validation Therapy (Feil, 1993, 2002). Box 9.2 provides a definition.

Box 9.2 Definition of Validation Therapy

A method of communicating with and helping disorientated very old people. It is a practical way of working that helps reduce stress, enhance dignity and increase happiness. Validation is built on an empathetic attitude and a holistic view of individuals.

'When one can step into the shoes of another human being and see through their eyes, one can step into the world of disorientated very old people and understand the meaning of their sometimes bizarre behaviour.'

Source: The Validation Training Institute Incorporated, online at https://vfvalidation.org/web.php?request=what_is_validation (accessed 10 November 2014)

This approach is based on respect and empathy. The carer, in recognition that the 'here and now' can often be painful and distressing for the person with dementia, interacts with the person in their world.

The validation approach is based on the following assumptions.

- That all behaviour has meaning. The way in which the carer responds to these behaviours and emotions can either increase their intensity or help to resolve them.
- The person will draw upon early emotional memories, learned from past life experiences, to replace intellectual thinking that may be lost.
- That older people with dementia will return to the past in order to:
  a) cope with the distress and painful feelings that so often accompany dementia
  b) allow them the opportunity to revisit the past and resolve unfinished conflicts
  c) relive positive past experiences and re-stimulate memories as a way of coping with current painful feelings and distress.

As an example, Box 9.3 introduces Mr Thomas.

Box 9.3 Introducing Mr Thomas

Read the following scenario.

Mr Thomas, a person with dementia, was standing in the main corridor of the ward looking quite agitated, pacing up and down, attempting to stop people that were passing him. A member of staff approached him and asked if he was OK and what was he doing standing alone in the corridor? Mr Thomas replied, 'I'm waiting for a bus to take me home. My wife will be worried about me.' The staff member replied, 'Oh that explains it. Well, don't worry, I expect one will be along in a few minutes.' Mr Thomas continued to stand and wait for the bus.

Imagine that you are observing this scenario, and consider the following:

- Was the staff member's response appropriate?
- How might a validation approach explain Mr Thomas's behaviour?

Discussion

It appears that the staff member recognised Mr Thomas's distress and agitation, and attempted to make him feel more relaxed by reassuring him that a bus would be along any minute. You might think that this was a well-meaning response, however it failed to alleviate the anxiety experienced by Mr Thomas. It is possible that Mr Thomas would become more agitated while waiting for a bus that is never going to arrive.

An alternative approach is to remember that all behaviour has meaning, and that it is important to try to empathise with Mr Thomas, to see the world through his eyes and become aware of his underlying emotions. Perhaps Mr Thomas is missing his home and family? His role of husband and provider has been gradually eroded due to the symptoms of dementia. While we may be unable to make it possible for Mr Thomas to go home we can give him the opportunity to validate his feelings and emotions by talking about how much he misses being home, and help him to remember the good times through past memories. This approach may alleviate his anxiety.

Using validation principles in this scenario you could:

- recognise that this is not really about a bus! Stand back and observe Mr Thomas for a few minutes and feel the underlying emotions that are being expressed through his behaviour.
- ask Mr Thomas what his wife is like, how long he has been married, and if he has any children. Help him to remember that he is a good husband.
- ask Mr Thomas if he is missing his wife today. Give him the opportunity to recall pleasant memories from the past to avoid the pain and distress experienced in the present.
- ask Mr Thomas if he has ever been apart from his wife in the past. If 'yes', ask him how he coped. Perhaps ask if he has, or would like, a photograph of his wife in his wallet.

The research is mixed when it comes to conclusions about the effectiveness of Validation Therapy. Although widely used in some areas of clinical practice there is insufficient evidence to support its effectiveness when used with people with dementia (Neal and Briggs, 2003). This does not mean that it is necessarily ineffective, instead indicating a lack of research into the uses and possible benefits of this approach. Many clinicians tell of anecdotal evidence of the effectiveness of validation techniques when working with behaviours that we find challenging as well as emotionally distressing. In our experience we have observed (and participated in) many instances in which validation techniques have worked effectively, along with some others where they have not.

Maintaining identity: meeting needs, feelings and emotions

In Box 9.4 you are invited to engage in an experiment.

Box 9.4 Being lost and confused

Imagine how it must feel to be lost in a foreign country, unable to speak the language used (receptive dysphasia). Think about not being able to find your way to the place where you are staying, and not knowing how to contact your family and friends (place disorientation). Imagine trying to explain to passers-by that you are lost, but finding that no one speaks your language (expressive dysphasia). You are unable to find your wallet or purse, so have no money or personal identification to hand (an inpatient on a dementia care ward). You are unable to follow directions and read the road signs (visual agnosia).

How would you feel?

This is a distressing experience and can easily happen to a person with dementia. This situation simulates some of the common symptoms of dementia (see Box 9.5) and will trigger feelings of insecurity, fear, frustration and anxiety, which will affect behaviour. For example, pacing and searching for familiar people or objects (wife, daughter, handbag), repetitive questioning, and becoming verbally or physically agitated. Through language we communicate our inner thoughts, feelings and desires, and herein lies the difficulty for the person with dementia. Therefore the carer must learn to 'step into the shoes' of the person with dementia and attempt to understand what the person may be feeling through their behaviours and the carer's knowledge of the person's life history. The challenge for the nurse is to draw upon an approach that enables them to develop a deeper understanding of the person's situation, feelings, values and thoughts so that the person's well-being is maintained and they remain connected to and engaged with the outside world.

Box 9.5 Common symptoms of dementia

- **Receptive dysphasia** is a difficulty in understanding spoken words.
- **Expressive dysphasia** ranges from difficulty in finding and expressing words or completing sentences to a complete inability to speak.
- **Visual agnosia** is the loss of the ability to recognise objects, faces, voices or places.

A prerequisite of the ability to apply a validation approach is having the right attitude towards the people that we care for. Christine Bryden, a person with dementia, sends a powerful message to her future carers when she writes:

> How you relate to us has a big impact on the course of the disease. You can restore our personhood, and give us a sense of being needed and valued. There is a Zulu saying that is very true, 'A person is a person through others'. Give us reassurance, hugs, support, a meaning in life. Value us for what we can still do and be … It is very hard for us to be who we once were, so let us be who we are now – and realise the effort we are making to function. (Bryden, 2005, p. 127)

Therapeutic skills that facilitate validation

Validation, in the general sense, can be considered as a kind of philosophy of care. It is identified as providing a high degree of empathy and an attempt to understand a person's entire frame of reference, however disturbed that might be (NICE, 2006, p. 387). It draws on the Rogerian humanistic principles of empathy, warmth and unconditional regard (Rogers, 1959) (see Chapter 3). The focus will be on applying these skills to people who are experiencing dementia; however the principles on which these approaches are based, and a number of these skills, can be applied to people with a range of mental health conditions. It is important to acknowledge that no single approach is suitable for everyone. The techniques used will depend on the individual, and before making a decision on which approach to use you should consider factors such as the person's level of cognitive impairment, his or her communication skills and comprehension abilities, and the individual preferences of the person. This will help to ensure that the care is both individualised and person centred.

In many other areas of mental health care there is now a strong evidence base to support the use of specific therapeutic interventions. Unfortunately, in dementia care this evidence base is far less robust. In the UK, the National Institute for Health and Care Excellence (NICE) guidelines for dementia conclude that 'there is no evidence that standardised approaches, such as validation, cognitive stimulation and reminiscence, reduce behaviour that challenges in people with dementia' (NICE, 2006, p. 230). However there is some evidence that these interventions can improve the person's well-being and quality of life (Neal and Barton Wright, 2009). What this means in clinical practice is that the approaches used are often based on informed trial and error. An approach that works well with one person may not work as well with someone else. It is therefore important to evaluate the effectiveness, or otherwise, of the interventions we use. It is also imperative that this information is communicated with the rest of the care team and recorded in the service user's notes. From our own experiences of working in dementia care, we have seen some excellent therapeutic approaches being used, but this information has often not been formally recorded and recognised. This is possibly due to the fact that these interventions are being used in an informal way as part of the day-to-day care of the person. All the skills that are going to be considered should be seen as being applicable to the normal daily routines in care settings. They do not require extra staff or resources, which are invariably in short supply.

Positive Person Work as a means of supporting validation

Psychologist Tom Kitwood has had a major influence on the way care is delivered, especially for people with dementia. Kitwood argued that the experience of dementia is unique to the individual and will depend on the interaction of many different factors. Positive Person Work concerns a range of interactions that will enhance a person's feelings of self-worth and well-being. Its aim is to place the individual at the centre of care, promote positive feelings and emotions, and help to retain abilities that would otherwise become lost and forgotten (Kitwood, 1997).

Kitwood outlined 12 types of interaction that aim to promote Positive Person Work.

1. **Recognition:** the person is acknowledged as being an individual by the carer, and respect is demonstrated through eye contact, personal greeting and actively listening.

2. **Negotiation:** the person is empowered and enabled to make choices, ask questions, consulted and listened to.

3. **Collaboration:** the carer recognises remaining abilities and provides opportunities that enable the person to participate in all possible activities.

4. **Playfulness:** this is about enjoyment and fun. The person's creativity is encouraged through activity and humour.

5. **Stimulation:** the senses are used as a means of communication – for example, using touch, massage, smell, aromatherapy, baking.

6. **Celebration:** enjoying each minute of each day, encouraging an overall feeling of well-being.

7. **Relaxation:** a recognition that people sometimes need calm and may need help to achieve this – for example, assisting someone to dress in a relaxed and unhurried manner.

8. **Validation:** acceptance of a person's reality and recognising the significance of feelings and emotions. Empathising with underlying feelings.

9. **Holding:** providing psychological support, 'being there' and responding to needs.

10. **Facilitation:** this follows on from collaboration and refers to the carer supporting the person to undertake a task that they may not be able to do.

11. **Creation:** being provided with opportunities to be spontaneous – for example, beginning to sing or dance.

12. **Giving:** the person offers gifts of affection and warmth to the carer, and this is accepted and reciprocated with gratitude and respect.

Maintaining personhood

Kitwood (1997) relates the concept of personhood to people with dementia and in doing so emphasises the need to value each individual as being a unique person with individual rights and needs. The social environment, in turn, can promote interactions that either maintain or destroy the personhood of the individual (Baldwin, 2010). Personhood 'is a standing or status that is bestowed upon one human being, by others, in the context of a relationship and social being. It implies recognition, respect and trust' (Kitwood, 1997, p. 8).

Continue to think about this in the context of a person who has dementia, taking account of the progression of stages of dementia defined by Keady and Nolan (1994) and summarised in Box 9.6.

Box 9.6 Nine-stage model of dementia

1. **Slipping:** where the person gradually becomes aware of minor and seemingly trivial slips and lapses in their memory and/or behaviour.
2. **Suspecting:** where memory lapses occur with greater frequency/severity so that they can no longer be rationalised or ignored.
3. **Covering up:** where the person makes a conscious and deliberate effort to compensate for their difficulties and actively to hide them from family members, friends and colleagues.
4. **Revealing:** is reached where the individual's difficulties are revealed to those closest to them. This may be as a result of a conscious decision, or as a result of being confronted with patterns of loss.
5. **Confirming:** is where open acknowledgement of the problem is made and the process of diagnostic conformation begins. This is usually the first point of contact with formal services.
6. **Maximising:** is where the person adapts by using coping strategies.
7. **Disorganisation:** is where the person experiences a diminished ability and awareness.
8. **Decline:** is where the demands of care increase.
9. **Death.**

Source: Gilliard, 2001

There are some very practical things that you can do to promote a person's identity.

- Find out about the person's life history. Most care facilities have biographical tools – for example, the recently developed This is Me, a tool for people with dementia who are receiving professional care in any setting that can be accessed via the Alzheimer's Society website (http://alzheimers.org.uk/thisisme). Ideally this should be completed with the person themselves, however if the person does not have the verbal skills and/or memory capacity to complete this then consider asking the people that know the person best, such as their family and/or main carers.

- Try to focus on what the person can still do and enjoy, rather than on what they are unable to do. For example, if the person has a poor short-term memory then asking questions about what happened recently may have no meaning or relevance to them, so rather than asking what they had for breakfast when you come on a late shift, ask about their working life – even though this may have been decades ago, it still has meaning to them. It is important to bear in mind that people with dementia will often revert to living in a time they can remember.

- Try to find meaning in the behaviour that people with dementia exhibit, rather than label it as challenging behaviour or behaviour resulting as a direct consequence of the dementing process. Kitwood (1993) suggests that this behaviour is an expression of an unmet need (comfort, attachment, inclusion, occupation and identity). For example, what might be labelled as 'wandering' could be a purposeful attempt to exercise or to try to find a way home. It may just be a case of asking the person where they are going that will provide us with the answer.

Reminiscence as a means of supporting validation

Recalling past events is a normal activity that we all enjoy participating in. School reunions, weddings and even funerals are all situations whereby we will often end up reminiscing with family and friends. Reminiscence can be particularly relevant for the person with dementia as short-term memories fade and long-term memories remain intact. The therapeutic value of reminiscing has long been recognised (Woods et al., 2005). Reminiscence can be used to activate communication, enhance well-being, strengthen individualised care and foster identity (Woods, 2002). Reminiscence provides an opportunity to share past experiences and meaningful life events with others. It facilitates social interaction and raises self-esteem, encourages verbal and non-verbal communication, stimulates past memories, and forges links between past and present. It highlights personal abilities as opposed to the things that a person can no longer do (Bruce and Schweiter, 2010). Reminiscence can also provide the carer with a different view of the person with dementia, and can be a reminder of who this person really is.

The terms 'reminiscence' and 'Reminiscence Therapy' are often used in the same context, but an important point to note is that Reminiscence Therapy is a specific technique that is delivered by suitably qualified professionals who are experienced in dealing with the possible distress and emotions that may be provoked. This chapter considers reminiscence as a means of supporting a validation approach. However, it is important to be aware that a reminiscence approach can arouse unexpected emotions and reactions, and where this occurs time must be spent helping the person to deal with them effectively.

Reminiscence can be used in many different ways.

• Books, pictures, photographs, videos, memory boxes that are age appropriate can be used as props to remind people of past experiences and stimulate tactile and visual memory.

• Rummage boxes or bags that include a range of tactile experiences. For example, items that relate to past occupations such as different fabrics for the dressmaker, tools and carpet cut-offs for the carpet layer and cookery utensils for the chef. These will need to be risk assessed with regards to being left in public areas.

• Work with individuals to develop life story books or personalised scrapbooks.

• Network with local museums and libraries as these may lend materials and support reminiscence activity.

Sensory approaches as a means of supporting validation

A key message throughout this chapter is that, for good-quality dementia care, it is essential that we see the person beyond the dementia and deliver care that is empathic and respectful. To do this we need to find a way to activate each individual's potential to communicate. We need to help the person be who they truly are, to know their likes and dislikes, their personality, and help them to use their retained abilities and potential.

In Box 9.7 you are invited to consider a question.

Box 9.7 Do you agree or disagree with the following statement?

As people enter into the moderate to late stages of dementia they are no longer the person they once were and it becomes impossible to communicate with and establish a relationship with them. The main focus of care must be to provide assistance with all aspects of physical care, and ensure that the person is nursed in a safe and respectful environment.

Discussion

As people enter into the more advanced stages of dementia it becomes increasingly challenging to show others who they still are, to express their thoughts, feelings and emotions, due to their decreasing cognitive abilities, impaired memory and communication difficulties. In our experience communication is always possible. A brief connection between two people can be expressed through eye contact, a warmness or recognition, and a smile of acknowledgment. A sensory approach will use a variety of experiences to stimulate all the senses (touch, taste, smell, sight, hearing) and movement, and aims to find a means of connecting with the person and overcoming the difficulties experienced at the moderate to late stages of dementia.

Sonas aPc (Activating the Potential to Communicate)

Pioneered by Sister Mary Threadgold, the Sonas programme is a therapeutic communication activity that focuses on stimulation of all the senses, in the belief that the senses are the gateway to communication. Benefits are varied and numerous. Please refer to the website for an in-depth analysis of its benefits: www.sonasapc.ie.

The End of Life Namaste Care Program for People with Dementia

Namaste is Hindu for 'honoring the spirit within' (Simard, 2013) and is an approach developed by Joyce Simard to provide carers with the means to connect in meaningful and engaging ways with individuals in the advanced stages of dementia. It aims to create a peaceful end to life, by reducing the anxiety and agitation that people with dementia may experience, through calming yet meaningful activity, comfort and pleasure.

The approach focuses on the person rather than the disease, and emphasises the enduring personhood of individuals despite the severity of the dementia. The Namaste approach focuses on the needs and spirit of each person through sensory-based practices that provide stimulation and relaxation: soothing music, light massage, gently interactive activities, familiar and pleasant smells, and a calming environment, all of which provide physical comfort and a loving touch to individuals who are too frail or cognitively challenged to engage in regular activity.

Conclusion

To treat people with dementia in a person-centred way we must first see them as people and not as a diagnosis and set of symptoms. This can be challenging if the care setting is orientated towards a medical model approach. It is nevertheless achievable with the right attitude. Try to think about how you or your loved ones would like to be treated if you or they were suffering from dementia.

Validation skills can be an effective means of delivering person-centred care. Central to the use of validation approaches is the ability to recognise and empathise with the person who has dementia and is experiencing the world differently from us. In order to understand the person with dementia it is important that we learn about them and what they were like before they had dementia. This helps to reinforce the concept of personhood.

Different approaches are required at different stages of dementia and it is important to tailor your approaches to benefit the individual. Bear in mind their communication skills, cognitive status (particularly memory), personality and personal preferences. Some of this information will come from cognitive assessment, but most will come from you getting to know them personally.

Most of the validation approaches discussed can be applied in your day-to-day care of people with dementia, and can also be adapted to the care of people with other mental health conditions in which cognition and perception are affected.

Activities

Activity 1

Reflect on what 'a person is a person through others' might mean to you. Relate this to a person with dementia.

You might have concluded that a person with dementia will experience a number of difficulties in representing the person they truly are. As the dementia progresses the nurse will play an important role in helping the person with dementia to maintain their identity and support them to remain the same person throughout the course of their dementia.

Activity 2

Consider Kitwood's 12 strategies for Positive Person Work. Which techniques did you observe being used while on placement or work experience? Which techniques did you use?

Activity 3

Consider reminiscence as a therapeutic tool. Think back to an event or a time when you reminisced. What did you reminisce about? How did you feel during and after the reminiscence? Was it an enjoyable or upsetting experience?

Suggested reading

Downs, M. and Bowers, B. (2014) *Excellence in Dementia Care: Research into Practice,* 2nd edn. Maidenhead: McGraw-Hill/Open University Press.

This book is interesting and informative, bringing together a wealth of expertise in dementia care to support best practice.

References

Alzheimer's Society (n.d.) Online at www.alzheimers.org.uk/ (accessed 13 October 2015).

Baldwin, C. (2010) Towards a person-centred ethic in dementia care: doing right or being good?, in Downs, M. and Bowers, B. (eds) *Excellence in Dementia Care: Research into Practice* (pp.103–118). Maidenhead: McGraw-Hill/Open University Press.

Bruce, E. and Schweiter, P. (2010) Working with life history, in Downs, M. and Bowers, B. (eds) *Excellence in Dementia Care: Research into Practice* (pp.168–186). Maidenhead: McGraw-Hill/Open University Press.

Bryden, C. (2005) *Dancing with Dementia: My Story of Living Positively with Dementia.* London: Jessica Kingsley Publishing.

Department of Health (2013) *Improving Care for People with Dementia.* London: Department of Health.

Feil, N. (1993) *The Validation Breakthrough: Simple Techniques for Communicating With People with Alzheimer's-type Dementia.* Baltimore, MD: Health Professions Press.

Feil, N. (2002) *The Validation Breakthrough: Simple Techniques for Communicating With People with Alzheimer's-type Dementia*, 2nd edn. Baltimore, MD: Health Professions Press.

Gilliard, J. (2001) The perspectives of people with dementia, their families and their carers, in Cantley, C. (ed.) *A Handbook of Dementia Care* (pp.77–90). Buckingham: Open University Press.

Keady, J. and Nolan, M. (1994) Younger onset dementia: developing a longitudinal model as the basis for a research agenda and as a guide to interventions with sufferers and carers. *Journal of Advanced Nursing*, 19, 4, 659–669.

Kitwood, T. (1993) Person and process in dementia. *International Journal of Geriatric Psychiatry*, 8, 541–545.

Kitwood, T. (1997) *Dementia Reconsidered. The Person Comes First.* Buckingham: Open University Press.

National Institute for Clinical Health and Excellence (NICE) (2006) *Dementia: Supporting People with Dementia and Their Carers in Health and Social Care.* London: National Institute for Clinical Health and Excellence.

Neal, M. and Barton Wright, P. (2009) Validation therapy for dementia. *Cochrane Database of Systematic Reviews*, 1.

Neal, M. and Briggs, M. (2003) Validation therapy for dementia. *Cochrane Database Systematic Reviews*, 3, CD001394.

Nursing and Midwifery Council (NMC) (2009) *Guidance for the Care of Older People.* London: NMC.

Rogers, C. (1959) *On Becoming a Person: A Therapist's View of Psychotherapy.* New York: Houghton Mifflin Harcourt.

Simard, J. (2013) *The End-of-Life Namaste Care Program for People with Dementia.* Baltimore, MD: Health Professions Press.

Sonas (n.d.) Online at http://sonasapc.ie/ (accessed 13 October 2015).

Woods, B., Spector, A., Jones, C., Orrell, M. and Davies, S.P. (2005) Reminiscence therapy for dementia (review). Online at http://onlinelibrary.wiley.com/doi/10.1002/14651858.CD001120.pub2/abstract (accessed 4 December 2015).

Woods, R.T. (2002) Non-pharmacological techniques, in Qizilbash, N., Schneider, L., Chui, H. *et al.* (eds) *Evidence-based Dementia Practice.* Oxford: Blackwell Science.

10

Preventing relapse

Iain Ryrie

Introduction

Helping people to prevent relapse after an intervention or programme of care is an important consideration for mental health nurses. A simple example is nicotine replacement products to prevent people relapsing to cigarette use. A more sophisticated approach is the use of family interventions among people diagnosed with schizophrenia to promote the 'emotional environment' within a family and thereby reduce the risk of relapse (see Chapter 16). There also exists an approach to counselling known as 'relapse prevention', and that is the focus of this chapter.

Relapse prevention (RP) is a self-management intervention to enhance the maintenance stage of a change process. Its primary goal is to address the problem of relapse and thereby generate techniques for preventing or managing its occurrence. Originally developed among people with alcohol problems, the RP model now provides an important framework for staff working with different service user groups, including people with a range of mental health problems.

This chapter introduces readers to the theoretical basis for RP, drawing on specific change theory and aetiological explanations for the development, onset and maintenance of a mental health problem. An overview of the service user groups and conditions for which the intervention demonstrates effectiveness is presented, followed by a detailed examination of RP practice skills for people with mental health problems.

Learning objectives

After reading this chapter, you will:

- understand the theoretical basis for RP and appreciate the hope this can bring to people with mental health problems

- summarise the purpose of RP and describe when it should be used to support an individual's change process
- describe the guiding principles and key stages of the RP approach
- understand how key stages of the approach are implemented in practice
- develop confidence in the use of some RP techniques in everyday practice.

Theoretical background

RP draws on many theoretical models and frameworks, two of which are central to understanding its value and application. The first is Prochaska and DiClemente's (1986) trans-theoretical model of change, also known as the 'cycle of change' (Figure 10.1). The model proposes that people pass through different

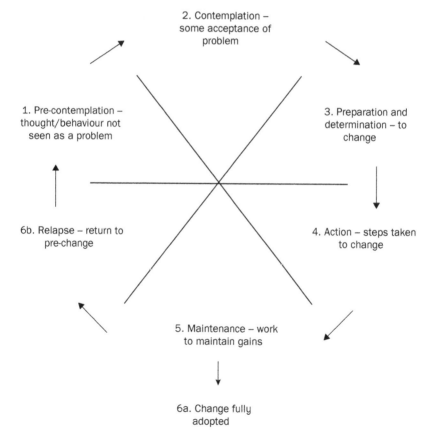

Figure 10.1 Cycle of change
Source: after Prochaska and DiClemente (1986)

stages when changing a behaviour or aspect of their lifestyle. If someone is trying to eat more healthily, stop smoking or adhere to a new meditation schedule, they will first need to make a decision to implement the change. There will then be some times when they are able to achieve their goals and other times when they waver in their actions. These events can be experienced as brief lapses, or they may herald a longer-term relapse to pre-change behaviours.

The cyclical nature of change can be seen in Figure 10.1. RP is used to support people in the bottom portion of the pie – the 'maintenance' stage of the change cycle. Most people who make an attempt at change will typically experience lapses that often lead to complete relapse (Polivy and Herman, 2002). This emphasises the value of an approach dedicated to supporting people in this stage of a change process.

The second theoretical basis for RP is Zubin and Spring's (1977) stress-vulnerability model, which explains the aetiology, onset and maintenance of schizophrenia, and is now used more widely to understand the development of mental health problems. Stress reflects the everyday pressures and concerns we all face, but also includes challenging life events such as bereavement, moving house or beginning a new job. A person's vulnerability is made up of different biopsychosocial elements such as genetic loading, cognitive functioning and social adversity. The interaction of these two components is presented in Figure 10.2.

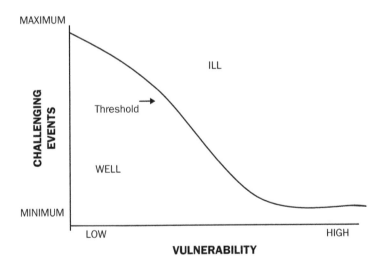

Figure 10.2 The stress-vulnerability model
Source: after Zubin, J. and Spring, B. (1977) Vulnerability – a new view of schizophrenia. *Journal of Abnormal Psychology*, 86, 103–126, reprinted with permission.

Zubin and Spring's (1977) key insight is that the dynamic interaction between an individual's vulnerability and the stress they experience in the course of their lives is the basis for the development of psychopathological symptoms. There is a range of vulnerabilities in any population, with some people being sensitive to crossing the illness threshold when experiencing relatively mild levels of stress. Conversely, others will have low vulnerability and can tolerate high levels of stress for significant periods without any trace of psychiatric symptoms. Illness episodes are also time limited, so that once any stress levels reduce below a vulnerability threshold the person returns to a pre-episode level of health.

An important implication of this model is the possibility of balancing our basic vulnerability and the stress we experience with protective factors in order to reduce the likelihood of relapse. For people with debilitating mental health problems, who may feel unable to control the occurrence of symptoms, this model offers hope. It suggests that interventions other than medication can be used to help them play a more active part in managing their illness. RP is an example of one such intervention. It is used to help people maintain any change by reducing the risk of relapse, and to equip them with knowledge and skills to manage any lapses to pre-change behaviour as and when these might occur.

Empirical evidence to demonstrate the effectiveness of RP has accumulated since the first randomised controlled trial among problem drinkers (Chaney, O'Learly and Marlatt, 1978). Studies have subsequently reported the benefits of RP for other service user groups, including those who experience depression, obsessive compulsive disorder, schizophrenia, bipolar disorder and panic disorders (Donovan and Marlatt, 2005). The approach is recommended in several guidelines produced by the National Institute for Health and Care Excellence (NICE), including guideline 38 on bipolar disorder. This recommends that RP is provided after an acute episode of illness to identify the symptoms and indicators of an exacerbation, and to make a plan for how to respond (NICE, 2006).

RP is a flexible intervention that can be used in multiple settings by staff with varying degrees of expertise. Given the potential benefit this could bring to people with debilitating conditions Sorensen, Done and Rhodes (2007) put forward a public health argument for treatments to be delivered by staff with relatively little training, using a limited number of sessions. In support of this argument, Sorensen has designed RP interventions for people with schizophrenia and bipolar disorder. In both cases mental health nurses, in partnership with their service users, are identified as potential users of these resources (Sorensen, 2005, 2006).

Sorensen's RP interventions comprise four 60-minute sessions, and have been published as brief treatment manuals and workbooks for therapist and service user (see the 'Suggested reading' section towards the end of this chapter). The material is designed to be delivered by expert and non-expert clinicians alike. Although few of us will have the inclination to become dedicated RP practitioners, it is possible to convey enough of the essential method to make it accessible, learnable and useful for developing practice skills. To assist this process, the case of Myra will be considered. Her experiences of RP are described throughout the next section, starting in Box 10.1.

Box 10.1 Case study: Myra

Myra is in her early fifties and lives alone in the suburbs after two previous marriages. She has one son who lives locally. By her late twenties Myra's behaviour had become increasingly unpredictable. Extended periods of frenetic energy coupled with soaring ambitions and confidence were contrasted with times when Myra couldn't lift her head from her pillow. Work became impossible and her first marriage ended. These fluctuating moods continued over the years that followed, sometimes with catastrophic consequences. At 35, Myra wooed her second husband by lavishing him with gifts while pretending to be a wealthy widow. Just days after a rapidly arranged marriage, and with tens of thousands of pounds of debt, Myra fell into a long depression. Her second husband eventually moved on, but not before he had spoken to Myra's GP, who initially made a home visit and then referred Myra to psychiatric services. Myra was diagnosed with bipolar disorder and, for more than ten years now, has taken mood-stabilising medication with varying degrees of success. Her last hospital admission was over a year ago, but she fully expects another at any point. Her son, who lives locally, does what he can but also keeps his distance, not just physically but in other important ways. He knows Myra can't help what happens to her so he doesn't expect too much from his mum and tries not to rely on her for anything. On the clearest of days, when Myra's mind is settled, she reluctantly admits to herself that she feels tattered and worn by this 'thing' her doctor calls an illness.

Practice skills

From these theoretical considerations it follows that the practice of RP is concerned with identifying high-risk situations in which individuals are vulnerable to relapse, and to help them develop strategies to prevent further relapses in similar situations. This section of the chapter offers some guiding principles for the practice of RP before breaking the process down into four key stages.

Guiding principles

RP is implemented in a spirit of mutual collaboration through which responsibility for the intervention is shared between the service user and the nurse. Person-centred counselling skills (see Chapter 3) form the basis of the intervention; these are tailored to guide the service user through the four-stage RP process. Sorensen (2006) has identified four guiding principles for the atmosphere and general style of an RP intervention, as follows.

1. **Express empathy:** use reflective listening skills to appreciate your service user's perspective and to communicate your understanding of it.

2. **Do not argue:** forcing your point through argument will spoil a therapeutic alliance and tends to generate resistance in service users. Offer alternative viewpoints with an open mind in the spirit of mutual exploration.

3. **Encourage self-efficacy:** many service users will need support to realise their ability to change or control some of their symptoms. However, Sorensen (2006) also emphasises the need to be realistic. Severe mental health problems are typically relapsing conditions for which one intervention is unlikely to solve all the associated problems.

4. **Use open-ended questions:** questions that avoid categorical answers such as 'yes' or 'no' encourage service users to engage and think more seriously about the matters under discussion.

Key stages

Although different practitioners may use different frameworks and language to describe their practice, RP basically follows a four-stage process (Table 10.1)

Table 10.1 The four stages of relapse prevention

Educate	To instil realistic hope in an individual's ability to have greater control over their symptoms
Assess	To raise an individual's awareness of their early signs, symptoms and triggers for an illness episode
Plan	How to react to any early signs, symptoms or triggers, and list the actions to take
Implement	Actions taken to balance or combat any emerging risks with protective factors

Educate

People like Myra can lack a belief in their ability to control the various symptoms they experience and hold negative expectations of how difficult life will be when symptoms recur (Sorensen, 2005). Their main contact with services may be to receive prophylactic pharmacological interventions interspersed with more intensive bursts of specialist input when medicines fail, or fail to be taken. Understandably, these beliefs and experiences can engender a sense of hopelessness in service users so it is important to help them develop an empowering and non-deterministic understanding of the nature of mental illness relapse.

Sorensen's (2005) RP intervention for bipolar disorder (BPD) achieves this by explaining the causes and influences of BPD with reference to Zubin and

Spring's (1977) stress-vulnerability model. Service users are encouraged to view their disorder as arising from an interaction between:

- biological factors (e.g. genetics and the effects of brain chemicals)
- psychological factors (e.g. hopes, expectations, interpretations)
- stress factors (e.g. a stressful job, financial difficulties, sleepless nights).

Activity 1

Reflect on your experiences of working with people who have mental health problems:

- what have they told you about the factors that contribute to the onset of an illness episode?
- what other factors have you noticed about their circumstances that may contribute to their problems?

Use Sorensen's (2005) biological, psychological, stress framework to organise your thoughts and write them down.

The aims of this educational component are twofold: to convey the potential to learn from what has triggered illness episodes in the past and thereby start to build up knowledge about stress factors that should be avoided because they increase the likelihood of illness; but also to view lapses as learning opportunities, from which further knowledge can be gained to adapt future coping strategies.

Box 10.2 contains a short excerpt of dialogue from Myra's first RP session, which is being delivered by her community psychiatric nurse (CPN), Cathy. She is visiting Myra at home and has just shared a simple handout with her that describes the stress-vulnerability model. The excerpt demonstrates the use of the RP guiding principles (these are shown within square brackets in the excerpt).

Box 10.2 Excerpt from Myra's first RP session

Cathy: So Myra, can you tell me what you make of these ideas that stress makes it more likely that a relapse will take place? [*open question*]

Myra: I'm not really sure – it's a bit like that chicken-and-egg thing, which came first? I would say the biggest stress in my life is my illness, which seems to cause most of my other worries.

Cathy: Yes, I can understand that and appreciate the problems your illness has caused you over the years. It's been very difficult for you at times [*reflective listening, expressing empathy*]. I wonder if it would be useful also to think about the times before an illness episode and your experiences of stress at those points – this handout suggests there might be clues at those times for why we become ill. [*not arguing, sharing an alternative view for consideration*]

Myra: That's funny cos, as you're saying that, I'm thinking about Bill, my first husband. He said he left me because I was mad, and I've always believed I became mad because he left me. So maybe there's something in it. I was very ill at that time and I always felt that my marriage breakdown and Bill's failure to support me made it all the worse.

Cathy: OK, that's interesting Myra. It sounds as though support from other people and harmonious relationships are important for your health. [*reflective listening, expressing empathy*]

Myra: I guess so ... but, hold on, are you saying that if I'd married the right man I wouldn't have had this illness?

Cathy: No, I don't think it's that straightforward. Let's look at this handout again. Illnesses arise from the interaction of all these factors, so no one thing, like a poor marriage, could be said to cause an illness episode. But it is possible to think about the different stressors in our lives, how they affect us and whether we can control some of them to lessen the impact of any illness. [*being realistic*]

Myra: And you think this could help me?

Cathy: I think you've already started the process. You've identified the importance of support from other people and harmonious relationships. We could do more of this work together and see what else we might learn? [*supporting self-efficacy*]

Assess

This stage of an RP intervention aims to raise service users' awareness of their early signs, symptoms and triggers for an illness episode. For BPD this needs to be undertaken for both depressive and manic episodes. Sorensen's (2005) programme includes worksheets for this purpose, with specific headings to prompt a service user's review of their illness experience.

Cathy is a creative CPN who took a flip chart and pens with her on her next visit to Myra. Once Myra had made a cup of tea they sat around the kitchen table with the flip chart in front of them. This is the process that Cathy took Myra through:

- The first sheet of paper already had three headings written on it: thoughts, feelings and behaviours. Cathy invited Myra to list under these headings any symptoms she experiences when she becomes depressed. This wasn't difficult to start with, but as Myra began to run out of ideas Cathy started to share other possible symptoms for her to consider and include in her list or not. Once Myra had listed all she could, Cathy asked her to underline those symptoms that she felt might be the first indicators of a developing illness.

- The second sheet of paper had two headings on it: positive events and negative events. This time Cathy invited Myra to list under these headings any stress factors that she believed had triggered an illness episode in the past. Again Cathy had some examples for Myra to consider, such as conflicts, losses, insufficient sleep and medication changes.

They repeated this process for Myra's episodes of mania and ended up with four sheets of paper full of ideas. Cathy offered to take them away and type them up. She returned them to Myra structured as a personal depression profile with triggers for her depression and, similarly, a personal mania file with associated triggers. Cathy invited Myra to check through the information, correct or add to it as necessary and, if possible, begin to think about whether it might be possible to combat or compensate for some of the triggers.

Plan
In this stage, service users are helped to identify personal criteria for when to react to changes in their illness profile and to list any protective actions they can take. The aim is to bring all they have learned together to create a 'relapse road map', or plan, for protecting their health in the future.

When Cathy visited again with her flip chart Myra had made some small changes to her depression and mania profiles, and they sat down to review them over another cup of tea.

- Together they looked at the early signs Myra had underlined in her profiles and their associated triggers. For each they thought about any strategies or actions Myra could use to try to combat the depression or mania, and listed them on the flip chart. Myra had already given this some thought before the visit and she had lots of ideas to begin with. Myra realised there was a connection between disturbances in her sleep and the occurrence of both manic and depressive experiences. One trigger was a habit she sometimes got into of watching TV endlessly through the night, dozing on and off but never sleeping properly. Myra felt she could do something about this. She also realised there was a connection between her illness and the frequency of contact she had with her son. The less she saw of him the more anxious she became and she wondered if this was one stress she could manage better.
- Cathy and Myra then created two simple plans from this work: one for when Myra was at risk of becoming depressed and one for when she was at risk of becoming manic. They included simple lists of important things to do and not to do, as well as the contact details of a trusted friend and mental health worker (Sorensen, 2005).

Once again Cathy agreed to take their work away and type up the two plans. They agreed to meet again in a month, after which Myra would have had time to implement some of her plans. Before ending this session Cathy congratulated Myra on the work she had done and suggested she review it regularly to become familiar with her illness profiles. Cathy also emphasised her belief in Myra's ability to carry out her plans, but was careful to point out that, if a lapse occurred, Myra could try to view it as a learning opportunity from which they could find better strategies for the future, rather than the beginning of an inevitable slide back into illness.

Activity 2

Activity 1 asked you to list the factors that have contributed to the onset of an illness among people you have worked with. Return to those notes and consider the following questions.

- Is there anything that could have been done differently to minimise the likelihood of an illness episode?
- What kind of support would your service users have needed?
- Who do you think could offer this support?
- How can it be maintained in the longer term?

Implement

People will need ongoing support to keep the RP process 'alive'. This is particularly true of people like Myra, whose previous experiences may have left them with a fatalistic sense of their illness, making it easy to slip back into old expectation patterns. Service users should be encouraged to develop and improve their profiles and plans. Sorensen (2005) considers these to be working documents that give people the opportunity to take more control over their illness than was previously possible.

Staff need to be available when lapses occur, maintaining a hopeful, realistic outlook, encouraging service users to view these events as learning opportunities. Box 10.3 contains a short excerpt of dialogue from Myra's fourth RP session, one month after her RP plans were developed with Cathy. Myra has had some success with improving her sleeping patterns and, although it's still early days, there were times when she felt calm and more centred than usual, but it hasn't lasted. More recently she met with her son and tried to tell him about her RP work. She didn't get very far as he wasn't responsive and at one point wondered if she was falling ill again. Myra lost her confidence, and since then has felt more anxious and less well. The excerpt demonstrates Cathy's attempt to make therapeutic use of this recent setback.

Box 10.3 Excerpt from Myra's fourth RP session

Cathy: Congratulations on making those changes to your sleeping patterns. It sounds as though they made a difference, but I can see how that's been outweighed by the difficulties you've encountered with your son. This is very important to you. Do you want to spend some time thinking about this problem and see if we can find a possible solution? There may be something important for us to learn from it.

Myra: Aren't we past that now?

Cathy: It may seem that way with some of the ideas we've had up to this point but I'd like to share another possibility with you, if you're happy to hear it.

Myra: OK.

Cathy: Family relationships can be some of the strongest influences on our mental health and I think that's what your experiences are telling us. What if we were to include your son in this programme in some way?

Myra: How exactly?

Cathy: I'm not sure, I think you're the best judge of that Myra, but here are a couple of ideas. We have factsheets on your condition that we could share with him to help him understand the different factors that influence mental health problems and how he may be able to help. That first session we had together, when we discussed the stress-vulnerability model, I'd be happy to share it with him and explain more about what you are aiming to achieve.

Myra: Really?

Cathy: Of course I would. We need to learn from what's happened and try something else. This could make a big difference for you.

Cathy did meet with Myra's son – on two occasions in fact. He came back after their first meeting of his own accord to share some ideas of how he could help his mum. Most months now he has a weekend meal with her and they share the responsibility for different courses. Myra feels more settled because of this and a little more secure. Part of her still expects a severe bout of illness to descend at any moment, but another part of her feels she's now doing something to protect herself from that risk. On her better days Myra calls this feeling her 'little kernel of hope'.

Conclusion

This chapter has introduced RP as an intervention to help people reduce the risk of relapse, while also equipping them with the knowledge and skills to manage any lapses to pre-change behaviour. In summary, the key points from this chapter are as follows.

- There is a dynamic interaction between an individual's vulnerability and the stress they experience in the course of their lives that explains the development of mental health problems.

- RP aims to balance our basic vulnerability and the stress we experience with protective factors in order to reduce the likelihood of relapse.

- People pass through different stages when making changes to their lives and RP is used to support people in the maintenance stage of a change cycle.

- The intervention is implemented in a spirit of mutual collaboration drawing on the guiding principles of person-centred counselling.

- RP follows a four-stage process:
  - educate to instil hope in someone's ability to have greater control over their symptoms
  - assess early signs, symptoms and triggers for an illness episode
  - plan how to react to early signs, symptoms or triggers
  - implement actions to balance emerging risks with protective factors.

- RP profiles and plans are working documents that should be reviewed regularly and refined with support from nursing staff.

Suggested reading

Sorensen, J. (2005) *Relapse Prevention in Bipolar Disorder: A Treatment Manual and Workbook for Therapist and Client*. Hatfield: University of Hertfordshire Press.

This is an invaluable text that presents the intervention in simple language. It is designed to be read directly to service users if staff do not feel sufficiently confident to deliver the content in their own way. It contains RP pro forma and handouts. The workbook is an excellent resource for service users. Sorensen's (2006) RP programme for schizophrenia and other psychoses is also available (see References).

Donovan, D. and Marlatt, G. (2005) *Relapse Prevention: Maintenance Strategies in the Treatment of Addictive Behaviours*, 2nd edn. New York: Guilford Press.

This text is written by the originators of the RP method and is an update of their original work. It is a valuable text for those interested in the wider applications of RP, e.g. among drug and alcohol users, people with eating disorders or gambling problems, but is more academic and less practice orientated than Sorensen's text.

References

Chaney, E., O'Learly, M. and Marlatt, G. (1978) Skill training with alcoholics. *Journal of Consulting and Clinical Psychology*, 46, 1092–1104.

Donovan, D. and Marlatt, G. (2005) *Relapse Prevention: Maintenance Strategies in the Treatment of Addictive Behaviours*, 2nd edn. New York: Guilford Press.

National Institute for Health and Clinical Excellence (NICE) (2006) *Guideline 38: Bipolar disorder: the management of bipolar disorder in adults, children and adolescents, in primary and secondary care.* Online at http://guidance.nice.org.uk/CG38/Guidance (accessed 12 March 2014).

Polivy, J. and Herman, P. (2002) If at first you don't succeed: false hopes of self-change. *American Psychologist*, 57, 677–689.

Prochaska, J. and DiClemente, C. (1986) Towards a comprehensive model of change, in Miller, W. and Heather, N. (eds) *Treating Addictive Behaviours: Processes of Change.* New York: Plenum.

Sorensen, J. (2005) *Relapse Prevention in Bipolar Disorder: A Treatment Manual and Workbook for Therapist and Client.* Hatfield: University of Hertfordshire Press.

Sorensen, J. (2006) *Relapse Prevention in Schizophrenia and Other Psychoses: A Treatment Manual and Workbook for Therapist and Client.* Hatfield: University of Hertfordshire Press.

Sorenson, J., Done, J. and Rhodes, J. (2007) A case series evaluation of a brief, psychoeducation approach intended for the prevention of relapse in bipolar disorder. *Behavioural and Cognitive Psychotherapy*, 35, 93–107.

Zubin, J. and Spring, B. (1977) Vulnerability – a new view of schizophrenia. *Journal of Abnormal Psychology*, 86, 103–126.

11

Behavioural management and activation

Geoff Brennan

Introduction

'Behavioural interventions' have often been portrayed as bad, if not evil. Books and films like *A Clockwork Orange* and *Brave New World* have so-called 'behavioural interventions' (shock therapy and social engineering) at the heart of their stories. These 'interventions' are being used to make people conform to some preconceived ideal of human behaviour. As people of free will we have an understandable aversion to being tampered with in the ways depicted. So, the discussion of behavioural interventions in this chapter starts with an axiomatic condition: behavioural interventions are always used to assist service users to achieve their goals. In other words, in modern mental health services both shock therapy and social engineering do not qualify as behavioural interventions.

Behavioural interventions in mental health are talking interventions. They are based on the assumption that our behaviour (i.e. what we actually *do* as opposed to what we *think* or how we *feel*) can be changed independently and that this change can overcome some of the difficulties we experience.

There are, of course, feelings and thoughts that will accompany a change in behaviour; often these will be thoughts like 'I can't cope with this' or feelings of anxiety or panic. Yet we can overcome these feelings and thoughts, and can change behaviour. If we look outside of mental health, behavioural interventions are used with people to help them stop smoking or lose weight. In other words, these are not interventions that are 'mental health' specific, but ones that can be, and are, used in a wide range of health and social settings – but always with the service user's full consent.

Learning objectives

After reading this chapter, you will:

- understand the principles of behaviour and operant conditioning, particularly in relation to depression
- understand the principles of functional analysis
- understand behavioural activation
- know the steps needed to carry out behavioural interventions
- have been introduced to social skills training.

As you will see, Box 11.1 invites you to engage in a first activity, involving thinking about things that make you personally anxious.

Box 11.1 The rewards of overcoming fear

Imagine something that makes you feel anxious. It could be a phobia, like spiders, flying or enclosed spaces, or an activity, like having to make a speech or undressing in a communal area. Whatever it is, make it real to you. Now imagine the things that would make you do this activity – the admiration of your peers, passing your course, a date with someone. Finally, imagine the feeling you would have once you have carried out the feared activity and achieved the deserved reward.

This process of overcoming a fear to achieve a reward is a frequent and common experience, but you can't overcome a fear of anything without confronting it. Many people you nurse will be paralysed by the feeling they can't do what they have just imagined, or are overcome with fear that they cannot achieve one of their goals. You have to believe they can. You can only do this by remembering that, while fear is common, so is overcoming it to achieve what we want. People do it all the time. The trick for many of us is finding something that's worth the effort.

Theoretical basis for behavioural interventions

Behavioural interventions primarily came about to assist people with depression and anxiety. In 1973 the American psychologist C.B. Ferster suggested depression could be seen as a way a person avoids or escapes from anxieties and fears in their life. This avoidance does not result in the person being happy as the pattern of avoidance or escape comes to be their main way of coping with their difficulties. As they get trapped into avoidance of activities to reduce anxiety, this also reduces their opportunities to do things that make them feel happy and fulfilled (Ferster, 1973). Hence, they become depressed.

Lewinsohn, Biglan and Zeiss took this further with a study of depressed and non-depressed people, which compared how often they engaged in 'pleasant activities'. The depressed cohorts were found to be engaging in fewer 'pleasant activities' (Lewinsohn *et al.*, 1976). The important thing about 'pleasant activities', as defined in the study, was that they were also seen to provide 'positive validation'. In other words, 'pleasant activities' feed in to a cycle of a person getting enjoyment by doing things that they perceive as worthwhile, and this in turn leads to them feeling fulfilled, engaged and useful. The avoidance of activities to reduce anxiety that was seen in the depressed person had the opposite effect – the avoidance made the person feel worthless and disengaged, and hence they felt depressed.

In the study there were thought to be three further reasons why a person experienced fewer 'pleasant activities' and less positive validation. Activities that had formerly been seen as pleasant and served as positive validation were less potent (e.g. a person who used to enjoy their job and get a great deal of satisfaction from it has now been in the job a number of years and no longer finds it as rewarding). Second, some activities were no longer available to the person (e.g. a person who used to go to the gym and enjoyed it had to stop because they were ill). Third, the activity may still be available but the person is no longer able to access it (e.g. a person who used to enjoy their church or a social activity is now too anxious to make the journey).

We can see from this that mental illness itself can contribute to the lack of 'pleasant activities'. People with mental illness are less likely to be employed or in relationships, and have a smaller social network than people who don't have mental health problems. In addition, they are more likely to be on long-term medication that comes with side effects and weight gain. Behavioural interventions have lot to offer people in overcoming these real and unwanted effects of a range of mental health problems.

Behavioural therapies try to do two things at the same time: increase the person's access to positive events while reducing their avoidance of anxiety. The difficulty is that, in order to get to the positive validation, they are going to have to abandon their use of avoidance, but the reason they use avoidance is to stop anxious feelings. So, in order to get to the positive validation, the person has to allow themselves to experience and overcome their anxiety.

Operant conditioning

Behavioural therapies are usually based purely on operant and respondent principles, aimed to change the service user's depressive mood by changing his or her behaviour patterns. (Shinohara *et al.*, 2013).

Operant conditioning postulates that people are more likely to repeat a behaviour if they are rewarded, or 'reinforced', for doing it. They are less likely to do the behaviour if they are punished for it. The following example presents a simple view of how we learn which behaviours are acceptable and which are not.

An example of reinforcement would be a child saying 'thank you' for something and a parent saying 'well done'. The behaviour is the child saying 'thank you' and the reinforcement (social praise) is the parent saying 'well done'. If the child values the praise and feels rewarded, they are more likely to say 'thank you' in future. An example of punishment would be a child pushing in to a line of children for a treat and a teacher making them go to the back. The behaviour is the child pushing in and the punishment is the teacher making the child go to the back (delay of the treat plus possible public humiliation). If the child views going to the back as an undesirable punishment for pushing in, they are less likely to do this in the future.

There is a complication in that, as well as the positive reinforcement described above, there is also negative reinforcement. Negative reinforcement is where a person is reinforced because the behaviour rewards them by taking away something they don't want rather than giving them something they do want. A classic example of both positive reinforcement and negative reinforcement is a child and a parent in a shop where the child is crying for chocolate and the parent eventually buys the chocolate to stop them crying. Here we would say the child is positively reinforced because they get what they want as a consequence of their behaviour. The parent is negatively reinforced because an unwanted desire is removed as a consequence of their behaviour. Table 11.1 shows the sequence in terms of:

- antecedent (what happens before)
- behaviour (what did the person do)
- consequence (what happens after).

Table 11.1 Antecedents, behaviour, consequences and outcomes

Reinforcement	Antecedent	Behaviour	Consequence	Outcome
Positive	Child wants chocolate	Child cries	Child gets chocolate	Behaviour more likely in future
Negative	Parent wants child's crying to stop	Parent gives chocolate to child	Child stops crying Parent feels relieved	

The child wants something it perceives as positive (chocolate), cries and gets it. This is positive reinforcement, as described above. The parent, however, has a crying child and wants the crying to stop. Giving the child chocolate stops this. This is called negative reinforcement as the behaviour (giving the child chocolate) is stopping something negative for the parent (the child crying). The outcome in behavioural terms is the same – both are more likely to do the same thing again in a similar circumstance.

The idea of understanding behaviour by looking at what happens before, during and after the behaviour is known as 'functional analysis'. Functional analysis allows us to consider how behaviour operates for the person and gives us some ideas as to how we can make things different. In the above example, if the parent feels guilty about buying the child so much chocolate we can look at a number of strategies to change the behaviour.

Evidence

The Cochrane Collaboration provides gold-standard analysis of the evidence behind any interventions and is used throughout the world to assess how good interventions are. A Cochrane Collaboration review in 2013 included a meta-analysis, which identified 25 trials of behavioural interventions used to treat depression. These involved 955 participants and compared behavioural therapies with other major psychological therapies (cognitive behavioural, psychodynamic, humanistic and integrative therapies). The analysis found 'low to moderate quality' evidence that behavioural therapies and other psychological therapies are equally effective. This really means that there is some evidence that behavioural interventions are as good as any other at helping service users with depression.

There is an obvious need for more research in this area, but the tools used in behavioural therapies are worth considering for a number of service users as the interventions really aim to assist service users to overcome anxieties in order to have a better quality of life.

A step-by-step guide to behavioural activation

Behavioural techniques are deceptively simple, yet they are difficult to put into practice as they deal with real people in real and powerful states of distress. As we discussed in the activity included in Box 11.1 earlier in this chapter, nurses have to really believe that service users can change their behaviour. Sometimes this belief can result in the nurse 'holding the hope' for a service user when they themselves do not feel they can achieve the change required.

We shall look at the stages of behavioural interventions, and use a simple example to highlight them:

- measure the behaviour
- monitor behaviour
- set objectives

- reinforce desired behaviour
- reduce incentives to perform undesirable behaviour
- evaluation and re-setting objective
- define behaviour that is the target for change.

When we realise something that is a problem for our service user, we can use functional analysis to get a better understanding of how it operates.

So, let's say we have John, who is on a ward and has not left his room since admission a few days earlier. When we talk to John he says he is very unhappy about being isolated, but he also had not left his flat for some weeks prior to admission. The only way he could cope with the journey to hospital was under heavy sedation.

We can start by asking him to tell us the last time he thought of leaving his room and what happened. This might look something like Table 11.2.

So, the behaviour that John experiences is 'being isolated in his room'.

Table 11.2 Working with John

Antecedent	Behaviour	Consequence
'John, tell me about the last time you wanted to leave your room. What happened?'	'So what did you actually do?'	'So what happened next?'
'Well, this morning a nurse came and told me my mother was on the phone and wanted to talk to me. I got dressed to go to the phone. I didn't make it.'	'I got to door of my room and imagined all the service users staring at me. I felt dizzy and scared, and lay on my bed. I could hear the noise of people outside and I felt sick.'	'After some time the nurse came back and asked if I wanted her to take a message. I said yes and she went away. I felt such a failure I cried. I stopped when she came back as I didn't want her to think I'm as pathetic as I am.'

Measure the behaviour

All behaviours are actions or 'doing' things that can and should be measured. Measuring gives the problem a shape and some structure. This should also be as simple as possible – e.g. how often does the behaviour occur or how long does it last.

In John's case, we could describe the behaviour in terms of time he is out of his room. We would measure time out of his room as we want John to experience a positive change, so the measure should go up as he spends more time out of his room. We could reframe this as a behaviour we want to reduce in which case we would measure time *in* his room. We would then see the measure go down.

Monitor behaviour

Once we have decided on a measurement, we need to make sure this is kept. The monitoring will be the focus for our discussion with the service user. In this way, we are both pooling our resources to see how we can improve outcomes against the measure.

So, for John, we would monitor the interventions by seeing if they are increasing his time out of his room.

Set objectives

Once the behaviour is defined, we also need to set objectives for the change we want. In doing this we should guide service users in making the changes SMART: **S**pecific, **M**easurable, **A**chievable, **R**ealistic and **T**ime-bound. For John, this could look like this:

- **Objective:** 'John will spend five minutes per shift (morning, afternoon and evening) in the day room over the next two days'
- **Specific:** this objective is specific as it states who (John), what (five minutes out of his room), and where (in the day room).
- **Measurable:** the measure is contained in 'five minutes per shift'.
- **Achievable:** John may have said a whole shift or a number of hours, but an initial change should be very small so that it is as easy to achieve as possible. We are looking for something that is achievable so we can build on the positives.
- **Realistic:** we are not asking anyone else to do anything and John does not need any special equipment. We could add a prompt for staff, but the general rule is the less complex the better.
- **Time-bound:** the two days means a total of six times (morning, afternoon and evening each day) before a planned evaluation. This means John won't be going for days feeling a failure or not being able to talk to someone to process what he has found.

Reinforce desired behaviour

It is very important that John be reinforced for any positive change in behaviour. If this can happen at the time, that is even better. So, if other staff notice him out of his room they could simply smile, or say how good it is to see him or offer him a cup of tea, anything, to increase John's sense of reinforcement.

Reduce incentives to perform undesirable behaviour

There will be many reasons why it is difficult for a service user to change behaviour. What we are trying to do here is to identify the mechanisms that give a service user permission to avoid or undermine the change in behaviour. This would require a little more negotiation with John as to how we can remove some of the things that are keeping him from facing his anxiety. An example is the kind nurse in our functional analysis interview who 'took a message' when his mum called. We could negotiate that it would be better if the nurse had asked his mum to call back so that he did not avoid the situation but had to confront it again. We could also find that other nurses are bringing his meals into his room when it would be better for John to at least attempt to collect his meal from somewhere and then go back to his room. All would have to be carefully explained so that John does not see changes as punitive and his basic needs are met – so, if he really cannot come out, a meal is brought to him and he is reassured that there is always another time to try to collect it.

This also highlights an important aspect of behavioural interventions: a consideration of the environment and how other people can feed in to the negative behaviour. As in our example, this can often be seen as caring for the service user, but in reality it keeps them from confronting their anxiety. This is often seen in families and carers, and sometimes we have to give people 'permission' not to care in such a way as to reinforce the negative behaviour. Of course, the same people can also be recruited to make sure that the person is reinforced for the positive change, so they would notice and praise any such change. What is crucial is that people who may be influential in the behaviour, such as staff, carers and even fellow service users, should be given as full an explanation of what is being planned as is needed to let them assist the change.

Reducing incentives is more understandable if we are trying to reduce behaviour. For example, if a service user identifies that they want to lose weight after coming out of hospital, then a reduction in having goods such as crisps and sugary snacks in the house will make it more difficult for them to get them. Generally, the harder it is to carry out behaviour, the less likely it is to happen. Putting blocks in the way of undesirable behaviours is a very useful addition to such interventions.

Evaluation and re-setting objective

This is the crux of the change and where the therapist's skill comes into play. First of all – a reality check – *most* service users will not experience behaviour change as a positive *even if* they have achieved their goal. John, for example, could start an evaluation with:

> Yes, I sat in the day room, but I felt worse. All the service users were staring at me and I know they all think I'm pathetic. When I got back to my room I was so relieved.

We should anticipate this and warn service users that when they begin to tackle behavioural change they are most likely to feel awkward, stupid, anxious or any number of emotions other than pleasure. The rewards are often delayed, and the service user will have to experience discomfort and anxiety before they are achieved. There is no avoiding this, but we must be sympathetic with the service user's annoyance and frustration.

Evaluation is also a chance to review the goal, take on any lessons learned, adjust and renegotiate. It is not possible to be too prescriptive about this here as many of the skills you have come across in other chapters will come into play. The main thing is to keep the conversation going with your service users, and not to be paralysed by their frustrations and lack of hope.

We should also be ready to reduce the objective to a smaller goal if it is too hard, and increase it if it is too easy. In many ways, behavioural change is never measured in terms of 'success and failure' but rather 'what worked and what didn't work'.

This whole process – identifying behaviours to change and getting people to overcome their anxieties to engage in more pleasurable activities – is called 'behavioural activation'. Box 11.2 contains a second activity, building on what we have learned about helping John.

Box 11.2 Working with John

Imagine that you and John have been working for some weeks now and there have been slow but noticeable improvements in the behaviour. John was spending ten minutes in the morning and afternoon in the day room and also longer at night in the lounge when most of the service users are asleep.

You are to evaluate the latest goal with John after what has been a difficult few days for the ward. A new service user was admitted who was in a manic state. In admission the night before, they saw John in the day room and tried to talk to him. John panicked and ran to his room where the service user followed and stood banging on his door until they were taken away by staff. Now, when John leaves his room, the service user instantly heads towards him.

What do you imagine the evaluation will be like? How do you think John will be? How do you think you should approach any objective planning?

A note on social skills training

One set of interventions often associated with behavioural interventions is 'social skills training'. This is a set of interventions that targets those with a serious mental health problem who have difficulties in interacting with others. In social skills training it is accepted that people with long-term mental health problems may have difficulties because they misinterpret other people's emotional responses or misread social signals. They may also have difficulty in interpreting what is the usual response in certain social situations. As a consequence they tend to stand out to others as 'different', not because of their psychotic symptoms but due to their social interactions.

Social skills training makes some assumptions. First, social competence (i.e. fitting in with others) is learned and not natural. We learn a set of social skills that make us socially competent. Social skills are therefore a set of learned behaviours (such as the child saying 'thank you' earlier).

Mental health problems get in the way of this learning, and can damage the social skills a person has learned. From this, dysfunction occurs when the behaviours are not in a person's repertoire. The behaviours are not used at the right time, and a person performs socially inappropriate behaviours (Bellack *et al.*, 2004). Social skills deficits can be overcome by training. This takes place in a group where people are taken through a set programme looking at learning social skills, rehearsing them and then carrying them out outside the sessions to see how they cope. The groups are run on behavioural lines in that they break the skills down and allow participants to learn how to adjust their responses. While this chapter is not aimed at describing social skills training in detail, it is worth noting that any such lack of social skills in service users is both well known and has a defined intervention aimed at assisting them to overcome the deficit.

Box 11.3 contains a further activity, again drawing on what you now know and on your experiences in practice.

Box 11.3 Putting it all together: behavioural interventions in action

Think of a service user you have met who has an identified social skill deficit. This could be someone who does not say please or thank you, is difficult to talk to because they interrupt you when you are talking, give you little feedback when you talk to them, end conversations abruptly or ask you overfamiliar questions. It could also be someone who stands out because they do not observe the 'social niceties'. Define the deficit you identify in behavioural terms, and design a set of instructions or interventions that could assist them with this.

Conclusion

Behavioural change is not confined to the treatment of mental health problems. The key to behavioural change is overcoming the blocks to activities that provide service users with long-term pleasure and validation. Service users can be assisted to change their behaviour through systematic measurement of behaviour and gradual movement towards a desired outcome. While the evidence is modest, the interventions can be useful in a range of situations.

Suggested reading

Veale, D. (2008) Behavioural activation for depression. *Advances in Psychiatric Treatment*, 14, 29–36.

This is a well-written, succinct article about behavioural activation that will further explain some of the points in this chapter.

Kuipers, E., Leff, J. and Lam, D. (2002) *Family Work for Schizophrenia: A Practical Guide*, 2nd edn. London: Gaskell Press.

Families and carers can help clients with behavioural change. This book outlines how this can be done.

Bellack, A.S., Mueser, K.T., Gingerich, S. and Agresta, J. (2004) *Social Skills Training for Schizophrenia: A Step-by-step Guide*. New York: Guilford Press.

As alluded to above, a very useful manual for those interested in social skills training – and it might help you with Activity 3.

References

Bellack, A.S., Mueser, K.T., Gingerich, S. and Agresta, J. (2004) *Social Skills Training for Schizophrenia: A Step-by-step Guide*. New York: Guilford Press.

Ferster, C.B. (1973) A functional analysis of depression. *American Psychologist*, 28, 857–870.

Lewinsohn, P.M., Biglan, A. and Zeiss, A.S. (1976) Behavioral treatment of depression, in Davidson, P.O. (ed.) *The Behavioral Management of Anxiety, Depression and Pain* (pp.91–146). New York: Brunner/Mazel.

Shinohara, K., Honyashiki, M., Imai, H., Hunot, V., Caldwell, D.M., Davies, P., Moore, T.H.M., Furukawa, T.A. and Churchill, R. (2013) Behavioural therapies versus other psychological therapies for depression. *Cochrane Collaboration Summaries*, 10. Online at http://summaries.cochrane.org/CD008696/DEPRESSN_behavioural-therapies-versus-other-psychological-therapies-for-depression (accessed 2 July 2014).

12

Mindfulness

Sali Burns and Steve Riley

Introduction

This chapter offers the reader an introduction to the application of mindfulness as a potentially transformative personal practice and as a therapeutic skill. An emphasis on a 'how to' approach will be provided, with an overview of relevant theory, and an exploration of relevant research and evidence for the application of mindfulness in the field of mental health nursing. Exemplars illustrating the skills utilised in mindfulness are included. The chapter will invite the reader to reflect on their own relationship and connectivity with the concepts and practices of mindfulness. It will conclude by highlighting the key features of the therapeutic approach and suggestions for further reading.

Learning objectives

After reading this chapter, you will:

- be able to discuss the theoretical basis for mindfulness as a therapeutic approach
- be able to reflect upon your experience, understanding and connectivity to mindfulness
- recognise the universal and specific application of mindfulness in the field of mental health nursing
- identify and report the research evidence supporting the application of this approach, and describe the benefits of the techniques
- be able to describe a step-by-step explanation of a mindfulness skill, illustrating the practical application of the approach
- know how to prepare and participate in a self-led mindfulness exercise.

The theoretical basis

Safe and appropriate use of mindfulness

In this chapter we suppose that the reader has little or no previous knowledge or experience of mindfulness. This being the case, we introduce the 'mindfulness' method, approach, therapy and way of life. In contemporary mental health services, all mindfulness-based approaches (MBAs) are centred on one of two programmes. The first, Mindfulness Based Stress Reduction (MBSR), was developed in the USA during the 1980s by Jon Kabat-Zinn and is described in his book *Full Catastrophe Living* (1990/2013). The second MBA used in mental health clinical practice is Mindfulness Based Cognitive Therapy (MBCT). This programme was developed by Zindel Segal, Mark Williams and John Teasdale in the 1990s for the purpose of preventing depressive relapse. The MBCT programme is presented in a week-by-week format in Segal, Williams and Teasdale's book *Mindfulness Based Cognitive Therapy for Depression* (2002/2013). In this book, they describe how the initial pilots of their depressive relapse prevention programme failed to achieve satisfactory results partly because the authors incorporated mindfulness only as a technique bolted on to a cognitive behavioural therapy framework. In reviewing and re-testing their programme, they found that, in order to learn the mindfulness skills that could help prevent depressive relapse, group participants had to be taught by mindfulness teachers who had a personal mindfulness practice. It was found the teachers embodied and modelled some of the key transformative factors of mindfulness – including an ability to resist the urge to fuel, fight or 'fix' when emotional distress was shown in the group. The learning gained from having a regular personal mindfulness practice enabled the mindfulness teachers to relate differently to their own distressing experiences. This meant they were able to encounter distress in the group in a 'mindful' way, which in turn helped the group participants learn that they too could relate differently to some of their unhelpful and distressing thoughts and feelings.

Earlier, Kabat-Zinn had also found it was necessary for the MBSR teachers to have an established mindfulness practice. Consequently, it is now accepted good practice for anyone wanting to teach mindfulness to have a 'commitment to a personal mindfulness practice through daily formal and informal practice' and the 'opportunity to reflect on/inquire into personal process in relation to personal mindfulness practice' (Implementation Resources, 2012).

If you think mindfulness has a potential role in your future nursing practice, we would like to guide you to begin the process of exploring mindfulness personally by:

- reading the MBSR and MBCT books introduced above
- attending an eight-week MBSR or MBCT course as a participant, not a trainee
- discovering how practising mindfulness can be (a) personally enriching and (b) personally challenging by establishing your own regular mindfulness practice – this will help you appreciate how much effort and commitment is

required of group participants when they are learning mindfulness as part of an MBSR or MBCT group

- finding a supervisor who has their own personal practice of mindfulness meditation, has taught at least nine MBA courses, has followed a mindfulness teacher training course at master's degree level and has attended a mindfulness supervisor's course.

Once you have found a supervisor, you can reach your own agreement on when and how you can integrate mindfulness into your mental health nursing practice.

For the foundation-level mental health nurse who is new to mindfulness, we therefore suggest that the information that follows should initially be used to help you decide whether mindfulness is appealing to you on a personal and professional level.

Background

The word *mindfulness* originally comes from the Pali word *sati*, which means having awareness, attention and remembering (Bodhi, 2000). Mindfulness as a concept has primarily been embedded in Buddhist traditions, with the aim of cultivating conscious awareness and the skill of being more aware of and attentive to what is happening to us in the moment. The key feature is the relationship between one's own attention and awareness with no separation between oneself and one's experience or activity in the present moment. Brown and Ryan (2003) described mindfulness as 'inherently a state of consciousness' that involves fully attending to one's moment-to-moment experience. Dictionary synonyms of mindfulness include alertness, diligence, carefulness, meticulousness and watchfulness, to name a few, whereas antonyms of mindfulness include apathy, laziness, thoughtlessness, lack of interest, ignorance and inactivity. The process of mindfulness has been described in various terms, such as meditation (Germer, 2005), reflection and reflective practice (Johns and Freshwater, 2005), and metacognition (Shapiro *et al.*, 2006).

Theoretical basis of mindfulness

The increasing interest and evidence base for the psychological construct of 'mindfulness' has led to research into the mechanisms of action underpinning the interventions (Shapiro *et al.*, 2006). Here we provide brief insight into the theoretical models offered, and encourage more in-depth additional reading for those with an appetite for theory.

Teasdale (1999) offers the theory that mindfulness contributes specifically to facilitating improved meta-cognitive insight, suggesting that, unlike cognitive behavioural therapy, mindfulness-based interventions work to change the mode in which cognitions are processed, thus increasing insight. Teasdale (1999) progresses the theoretical perspective and offers a conceptual framework:

interacting cognitive subsystems (ICS). The analysis of ICS suggests that differences between higher-order 'meta-cognitive' *knowledge* and meta-cognitive *insight* alter emotional meaning and emotional processing. Shapiro *et al.* (2006), in explaining the 'how does it work' question, suggest a model of mindfulness that includes three components (Axioms): *intention, attention* and *attitude* (see later in the chapter for examples). Shapiro *et al.* (2006) also introduce the notion of the meta-mechanism of action called 're-perceiving', which contributes to the transformational effects of mindfulness. In recent studies, functional and structural neuro-imaging have explored the neuro-scientific processes underpinning mindfulness theory. Holzel *et al.* (2011) report evidence which suggests that mindfulness in practice contributes to synergistic neural processes and is associated with neuro-plastic changes in the anterior cingulate cortex, insula, temporo-parietal junction, fronto-limbic network, and default mode network structures resulting in enhanced self-regulation.

Therapeutic benefits of mindfulness

We have said that MBAs were originally developed for use with stress and depression. Recent developments have seen the approach used with other mental health populations including people with substance misuse problems and eating disorders, among others.

Research projects across the world have helped confirm that mindfulness can improve quality of life, reduce distress and maintain mental well-being (Baer, 2003). Research has also started to isolate the elements of mindfulness-based approaches that bring about therapeutic change and how that might happen. Treadway and Lazar (2009, cited in Didonna, 2009) report that the clinical implications of practising meditation and mindfulness are an increased amount of time spent 'living in the moment', increased positive affect, reduced stress reactivity and enhanced cognitive vitality. Baer (2003) found that these changes may be due to the fact that mindfulness practices:

- involve repeated exposure to 'undesirable' sensations using a non-judgemental attitude
- bring about cognitive change by leading participants to understand that problematic thoughts are 'just thoughts' (Kabat-Zinn, 1982, 1990/2013, cited in Baer, 2003) and that 'the non-judgmental, decentered view of one's thoughts ... may interfere with ruminative patterns believed to be characteristic of depressive episodes' (Nolen-Hoeksema, 1991; Teasdale, Segal and Williams, 1995; Teasdale, 1999) influence self-management through improved self-observation, which leads to accessing a broader range of coping skills
- can induce relaxation – although Baer (2003) reminds us that 'the purpose of mindfulness training is not to induce relaxation, but instead to teach non-judgmental observation of current conditions, which might include

autonomic arousal, racing thoughts, muscle tension, and other phenomena incompatible with relaxation'

● cultivate acceptance by 'experiencing events fully and without defence, as they are' (Hayes, 1994, cited in Baer, 2003).

Williams and Kuyken (2012) say that:

> Unlike cognitive therapy, the mindfulness approach does not try to change the content of negative thinking. Rather, it encourages participants to change their relationship to thoughts, feelings and body sensations, so that they have an opportunity to discover that these are fleeting events in the mind and the body that they can choose to engage with – or not. That is, repeated practice in noticing, observing with curiosity and compassion, and shifting perspective helps participants to realise that their thoughts, emotions and sensations are just thoughts, emotions and sensations, rather than 'truth' or 'me'. They learn to see more clearly the patterns of the mind, and to recognise when mood is beginning to dip without adding to the problem by falling into analysis and rumination – to stand on the edge of the whirlpool and watch it go round, rather than disappearing into it.

A further description of how mindfulness can facilitate therapeutic change is given in Williams and Penman (2011). In mindfulness, the emphasis is on stepping out of a driven 'doing' mode of thinking and behaving, and entering a 'being' mode that involves inhabiting the body and neutrally observing current thoughts, sensations and emotions as they arise and pass away. Williams and Penman (2011) list the seven sets of 'doing' and 'being' modes of mind and show how – through mindfulness – we aim to move along from the 'doing' to the 'being' state. This is illustrated in Box 12.1.

Box 12.1 'Doing' and 'being'

'Doing'	'Being'
Automatic pilot	Conscious choice
Analysing	Sensing
Striving	Accepting
Seeing thoughts as solid and real	Seeing thoughts as mental events
Avoidance	Approaching
Mental time travel	Remaining in the present moment
Depleting activities	Nourishing activities

Evidence base

The evidence base for mindfulness has been developing in line with the rate of popularity of the approach. Davis and Hayes (2011) suggest that the success of MBSR programmes and the central role of mindfulness in dialectical behaviour therapy (DBT) (Linehan, 1993), and in 'acceptance and commitment therapy', have contributed to moving mindfulness from 'a largely obscure Buddhist concept to a mainstream psychotherapy construct'. Davis and Hayes (2011) report a plethora of theorised benefits of the approach, including self-control, objectivity, affect tolerance, enhanced flexibility, improved concentration, emotional intelligence, and the ability to relate to others and oneself with kindness and compassion.

Didonna (2009) and Shapiro and Carlson (2009) have reported on the effectiveness of mindfulness in physical or mental health settings – for example, MBSR for people suffering from chronic pain (Kabat-Zinn et al., 1987) and people diagnosed with cancer (Carlson and Garland, 2005). Mindfulness has been identified as helpful for people who experience hearing voices; Chadwick (2006) suggests mindfulness can help people learn to 'turn down' their experiences of the voices. The worrying increased cost to individuals and society due to depression has been identified worldwide and has been the subject of numerous studies. The benefits of dialectical behaviour therapy outlined by Linehan (1993) have been built upon by Lynch (2011), who describes the benefits of an adapted DBT programme for treatment-resistant depression, which includes the importance of increasing individuals' core mindfulness. As described earlier in this chapter, Segal et al. (2002/2013) developed MBCT for people who had suffered three or more episodes of depression, and demonstrated the effectiveness of reducing relapse in this service user group. In addition to treating physical and mental illness, interest has been growing in mindfulness as a way of increasing older people's positivity, reminding them of their inner strength, resilience and resources (McBee, 2008). Findings by Gallegos et al. (2013) suggest that MBSR improves positive affect for older adults with lower depressive symptom severity.

Mindfulness practice

Mindfulness develops the skill to direct our attention deliberately. Much of our waking time is spent in a state of automatic pilot, during which our attention wanders according to the whims of our internal thinking processes or in reaction to constantly changing stimuli in our environment. We often find that we get alerted to discomfort, pain, distress, pleasure or enjoyment only when they are sufficiently powerful to snap us out of our dreamlike state. Mindfulness helps us notice when things are OK as well as when they are not. Mindfulness enables us to turn on our attention when we are subtly aware of stimuli as well as when the stimulus is strong.

Mindfulness achieves this by enabling us to become more aware and in tune with our sensing self. We develop the discipline to use the physical senses of touch, sight, smell and taste, along with the sensing mind by engaging in formal and informal mindfulness practices. Formal mindfulness practice involves setting aside time to sit and follow mindfulness practices such as the body scan, mindfulness of breath, mindful movement and sitting meditation. Informal mindfulness is practised when we bring an attitude of mindfulness to everyday activities such as doing household tasks or eating.

Step-by-step explanation

In this section we are going to consider how mindfulness can be used in practice. Kabat-Zinn (1994) has described mindfulness as 'paying attention in a particular way: on purpose, in the present moment, and non-judgmentally' Shapiro *et al.* (2006) have interpreted these building blocks of mindfulness as the 'Three Axioms of Mindfulness' shown in Figure 12.1.

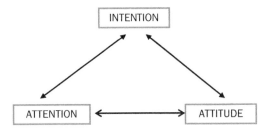

Figure 12.1 The Three Axioms of Mindfulness

In the following exercise we invite you to experientially explore this basic definition of mindfulness by following the instructions given.

Step 1: intention and attention

Without changing your posture, we would like to invite you to pause and then – when you are ready – begin to explore what is being experienced in your body at this moment. You may choose to pay attention by scanning your body from toes to head, or you might decide to sit quietly and allow any sensory information from the body to simply flow into your conscious awareness. Then, when you are ready, move the focus of attention away from the body and towards the mind, towards thoughts. You may notice that the mind is very busy and has many thoughts, or it may be very still in this moment. You may even find that there is nothing in particular for your attention to notice at this time.

Continue to do this over at least 60 seconds.

Step 2: attention

It is possible that your attention will drift away from focusing on the body or the mind during this exercise. Each time you become aware that this has occurred, just note that this has happened and bring the attention back to the focus of this exercise, which is to investigate what is being experienced in the body and in the mind at this moment.

Step 3: attitude

You may be aware of tension or relaxation, warmth or coolness in the body. You may be aware of the mind having thoughts that wonder about the future or worry about the past. Bring an attitude of acceptance, curiosity and non-judgement to whatever you encounter in the body and the mind. You may be aware of a desire to push unpleasant thoughts or feelings away, or of an urge to judge sensations in the body and thoughts in the mind as 'good' or 'bad'. Be curious about your experiences and your reactions. Accept things as they are in this moment. Bring a neutral, non-judgemental attitude to what you encounter.

Reflection

Now that you have followed this brief mindfulness exercise, please reflect on your personal experience of having followed these instructions.

- Were there any parts of the exercise that were easy to follow? What made these parts easy for you?
- Were there any parts of the exercise that were difficult to follow? What made these parts difficult for you?
- What was it like for you when you tried to bring an attitude of curiosity, acceptance and non-judgement to what was being felt in the body and being thought in the mind?
- How are you feeling now that you have completed this exercise? If you have experienced difficult thoughts, feelings or sensations as a result of following the exercise, ask yourself if you need to take some time to reflect on this before continuing with reading this chapter.

Next, we would like you to consider what it might be like for a person who has negative or anxious thinking to follow the above mindfulness exercise.

- What might be easy to do?
- What might be difficult to do?
- What might it be like for the person who has negative or anxious thinking to try to bring an attitude of curiosity, acceptance and non-judgement to whatever they might be experiencing in that moment?

- Would the mindfulness practice be more likely to make the person with negative or anxious thinking feel better or worse?

It is clear to practitioners and teachers of mindfulness that practising mindfulness can initially make things worse for the participant. During mindfulness practices, participants come up against the very things they spend time and energy trying not to feel or to think. In some ways this mindfulness practice can seem counterintuitive. Why on earth would we want to expose ourselves to the sensations, feelings and thoughts that cause us so much suffering? In normal circumstances, it is not always a good idea to get up close to troubling thoughts and feelings as they have a tendency to intensify and magnify under obsessive scrutiny. However, in mindfulness practice, we train ourselves not only to notice the difficult but also the pleasurable and the neutral. We also train ourselves to approach our experiences with acceptance, curiosity and kindness, and non-judgementally. The purpose of becoming skilled in paying attention to all our experiences, whatever they may be, is to help us make wise judgements and decisions, and to know when we can let go of worries and ruminations. We may live our lives in terror of the snake in the shadows, but when we turn the light of our conscious attention towards it, we often find that what we thought to be a venomous reptile is after all a coiled piece of rope.

Box 12.2 introduces you to Gwen, and shows the application of mindfulness in practice.

Box 12.2 Mindfulness in practice

Gwen has recovered from a depressive episode and has been following the MBCT eight-week course. She is now on session seven. The group is discussing how their home practice went.

> *Gwen:* I got a text from the team captain on Sunday to let me know my son's under-14s rugby game had been cancelled because the pitch was too wet. I started to feel upset because I was staying at my mother's with my two younger children and had only let my son go to his father's because of the rugby match. Because of feeling upset, I decided to do the coping three-minute breathing space. So I did it and it was good because I realised that my mind was going off – I was thinking that my son hadn't seen his gran in a while so it was a big deal for me to let him go to his dad's. Also, I was thinking about the fact that he only ever plays computer games at his dad's. It was making me feel bad. So I focused down on the breath and then expanded the focus out again at the end and felt better.

Mindfulness teacher: You had checked in to see what was happening in your mind at the beginning of the three-minute breathing space. Did you also notice how your body was feeling at that time, Gwen?*

Gwen: Yes. I had a heavy feeling in the pit of my stomach and I was feeling annoyed.

Mindfulness teacher: Where were you feeling the annoyed feeling in your body?**

Gwen: [*after a pause for thought*] In the back of my shoulders.

Mindfulness teacher: How did you respond to these sensations in your body, Gwen?

Gwen: Well, I was more aware of the heaviness in the pit of my stomach. I think I only realised now that I had that annoyed feeling in my shoulders too. The feeling in my stomach is something I've had before. It's something I dread, actually. But I decided to let it be there and thought I would just get on with the breathing space.***

Mindfulness teacher: What did you notice in your body during the focus on breathing?

Gwen: I found it quite easy really to just pay attention to the breath and not get distracted by any other feelings in my body.

Mindfulness teacher: When you expanded your focus again, what was that like?

Gwen: Well, the feeling in my stomach was there a bit, but because the thoughts that would have made it worse had dissolved, I was able to cope with having the feeling until it just went away.

Mindfulness teacher: Your troubling thoughts had dissolved?

Gwen: Yes, because I had stopped focusing on them, and concentrated on the breath and on my body instead, they just sort of went away.

Mindfulness teacher: So you found the three-minute breathing space helped you cope better?

Gwen: Yes, because at the end of the day, I had let my son go to his dad's for the rugby but there was nothing I could do about the game being cancelled. I just had to accept it. I want to support my son with his rugby but another time I might ask him to come with me to his gran's even if there is a game on because he loves his gran and it's important that he gets a chance to spend time with her.

Intention: The teacher is finding out whether Gwen started the practice by observing only her thoughts rather than thoughts, bodily sensations and emotions.

Attention: Gwen has stopped at labelling a body feeling 'annoyed'. The teacher is guiding Gwen to pay attention to what was actually occurring in the body, instead of just naming it.

***Acceptance:** Gwen has already been practicing mindfulness daily for several weeks and is learning that she does not have to react automatically to thought and sensations – even unpleasant ones.

Conclusion

Increasing mindfulness can positively contribute to preventing relapse in depression, and can promote emotional intelligence and our ability to relate to others with kindness. Mindfulness aims to cultivate conscious awareness and the skill of being more aware of and attentive to what is happening in the moment. Research projects across the world have helped confirm that mindfulness can improve quality of life, reduce distress and maintain mental well-being. As an approach, mindfulness emphasises the stepping away from the 'doing' mode of thinking and entering a 'being' mode. Data suggest that mindfulness-based interventions are effective for treatment of both psychological and physical symptoms. MBSR improves positive affect for older adults with lower depressive symptom severity. Mindfulness helps us notice when things are OK as well as when they are not.

We hope that the introduction to mindfulness in this chapter assists you to consider mindfulness as moving from an alternative therapeutic approach to a more mainstream one, and inspires an interest that will commence a journey of developing skills for future practice.

Activity

Mindfulness activity

Box 12.3 contains an opportunity for you to consider whether and in what ways personal and regular mindfulness practice could help mental health nurses:

1. provide care for mental health service users
2. care for their own psychological well-being
3. prevent burnout.

Box 12.3 Mindfulness activity

With a peer group of mental health students, listen to a mindfulness practice such as the Chocolate Meditation (http://franticworld.com/free-meditations-from-mindfulness/) and discuss your experiences of having participated in the practice.

Watch Jon Kabat-Zinn lead a session on mindfulness, on YouTube (www.youtube.com/watch?v=3nwwKbM_vJc).

Watch Bill Moyers' 1993 documentary *Healing and the Mind*, which shows interviews with participants from Jon Kabat-Zinn's MBSR course in the USA (http://vimeo.com/39767361).

Suggested reading

Kabat-Zinn, J. (2013) *Full Catastrophe Living: Using the Wisdom of Your Body and Mind to Face Stress, Pain and Illness*. New York: Dell Publishing.
This book is designed to help readers develop meditation practices, and to use mindfulness in everyday life.
Teasdale, J., Williams, M. and Segal, Z.V. (2014) *The Mindful Way Workbook*. London: Guilford Press.
This is a practical, step-by-step guidebook.

References

Baer, R. (2003) Mindfulness training as a clinical intervention: a conceptual and empirical review. *American Psychological Association*, 10, 125–143.
Bodhi, B. (2000) *A Comprehensive Manual of Adhidhamma*. Seattle, WA: BPS Pariyatti Editions.
Brown, K.W. and Ryan, R.M. (2003) The benefits of being present: mindfulness and its role in psychological well-being. *Journal of Personality and Social Psychology*, 84, 4, 822–848.
Carlson, L.E. and Garland, S.N. (2005) Impact of mindfulness-based stress reduction (MBSR) on sleep, mood, stress and fatigue symptoms in cancer outpatients. *International Journal of Behavioural Medicine*, 12, 4, 278–285.
Chadwick, P. (2006) *Person-based Cognitive Therapy for Distressing Psychosis*. Chichester: John Wiley & Sons
Davis, D.A. and Hayes, J.A. (2011) What are the benefits of mindfulness? A practice review of psychotherapy-related research. *Psychotherapy*, 48, 2, 198–208.
Didonna, F. (ed.) (2009) *Clinical Handbook of Mindfulness*. New York: Springer.
Gallegos, A.M., Hoerger, M., Talbot, N.L., Moynihan, J.A. and Duberstein, P.R. (2013) Emotional benefits of mindfulness-based stress reduction in older adults: the moderating roles of age and depressive symptom severity. *Aging Mental Health*, 17, 7, 823–829.
Germer, C.K. (2005) Mindfulness. What is it? What does it matter?, in Germer, C.K., Siegel, R.D. and Fulton, P.R. (eds) *Mindfulness and Psychotherapy* (pp.3–27). New York: Guilford Press.
Hayes, S.C. (1994) Content, context, and the types of psychological acceptance, in Hayes, S.C., Jacobson, N.S., Follette, V.M. and Dougher, M.J. (eds) *Acceptance and Change: Content and Context in Psychotherapy* (pp.13–32). Reno, NV: Context Press.
Holzel, B.K., Lazar, S.W., Gard, T., Schuman-Olivier, Z., Vago, D.R. and Ott, U. (2011) How does mindfulness meditation work? Proposing mechanisms of action from conceptual and neutral perspectives. *Perspectives on Psychological Science*, 6, 6, 537–559.
Implementation Resources (2012) Mindfulness-based cognitive therapy (MBCT). Online at http://mindfulnessteachersuk.org.uk/pdf/MBCTImplementationResources.pdf (accessed 4 December 2015).
Johns, C. and Freshwater, D. (2005) *Transforming Nursing through Reflective Practice*. Oxford, UK: Blackwell Publishing.
Kabat-Zinn, J. (1982) An outpatient program in behavioral medicine for chronic pain patients based on the practice of mindfulness meditation: theoretical considerations and preliminary results. *General Hospital Psychiatry*, 4, 33–47.

Kabat-Zinn, J. (1990/2013) *Full Catastrophe Living: Using the Wisdom of Your Body and Mind to Face Stress, Pain and Illness*. New York: Dell Publishing.

Kabat-Zinn, J. (1994) *Wherever You Go, There You Are: Mindfulness Meditation in Everyday Life*. New York: Hyperion.

Kabat-Zinn, J., Lipworth, L., Burney, R. and Sellers, W. (1987) Four-year follow-up of a meditation-based program for the self-regulation of chronic pain: treatment outcomes and compliance. *Clinical Journal of Pain*, 2, 159–173.

Linehan, M. (1993) *Cognitive Behavioral Treatment of Border-line Personality Disorder*. New York: Guilford Press.

Lynch, T.R. (2011) Dialectical behaviour therapy (DBT) for treatment-resistant depression (TRD): a randomised controlled trial (RCT). Online at www.nets.nihr.ac.uk/__data/assets/pdf_file/0004/54805/PRO-09-150-12.pdf (accessed 4 December 2015).

McBee, L. (2008) *Mindfulness-based Elderly Care*. New York: Springer.

Nolen-Hoeksema, S. (1991) Responses to depression and their effects on the duration of depressive episodes. *Journal of Abnormal Psychology*, 100, 569–582.

Segal, Z.V., Williams, J.M. and Teasdale, J.D. (2002/2013) *Mindfulness-based Cognitive Therapy for Depression: A New Approach to Preventing Relapse*. New York: Guilford Press.

Shapiro, S. and Carlson, L.E. (2009) *The Art and Science of Mindfulness: Integrating Mindfulness into Psychology and the Helping Professions*. Washington, DC: American Psychological Association.

Shapiro, S., Carlson, L., Austin, J. and Freedman, B. (2006) Mechanisms of mindfulness. *Journal of Clinical Psychology*, 62, 3, 373–386.

Teasdale, J.D. (1999) Metacognition, mindfulness, and the modification of mood disorders. *Clinical Psychology and Psychotherapy*, 6, 146–155.

Teasdale, J.D., Segal, Z.V. and Williams, M.G. (1995) How does cognitive therapy prevent depressive relapse and why should attentional control (mindfulness training) help? *Behaviour Research and Therapy*, 33, 25–39.

Treadway, M.T. and Lazar, S.W. (2009) The neurobiology of mindfulness, in Didonna, F. (ed.) *Clinical Handbook of Mindfulness*. New York: Springer.

Williams, J.M.G. and Kuyken, W. (2012) Mindfulness-based cognitive therapy: a promising new approach to preventing depressive relapse. *British Journal of Psychiatry*, 200, 359–360.

Williams, M. and Penman, D. (2011) *Mindfulness: A Practical Guide to Finding Peace in A Frantic World*. London: Hachette Digital.

13

De-escalating volatile situations

Elizabeth Bowring-Lossock

Introduction

Ensuring a safe therapeutic working environment for nurses and service users concerns all involved in the provision of health care (Health and Safety Executive, 1974; Royal College of Nursing, 2008). In the UK, guidance on the short-term management of violence and physically aggressive behaviour emphasises the importance of maintaining safety and well-being, highlighting the need for de-escalation of volatile situations through the use of excellent communication skills (NICE, 2015). All four governmental bodies across the UK support these principles in the context of rigorous clinical risk assessment and management, recognising that this is key to providing excellence in care delivery throughout mental health services (Department of Health, Social Services and Public Safety in Northern Ireland, 2007; Welsh Government, 2010; Department of Health, 2011; Scottish Government, 2012). Recent guidance advocates that 'Positive Behaviour Support' must include strategies to minimise and manage conflict, and that de-escalation must be formally care planned, and ensure that respect and dignity are maintained for all concerned (Department of Health, 2014).

People who are suffering from mental health disorders may on occasion be volatile and unpredictable, and may demonstrate verbal or physical aggression as a result. This phenomenon in inpatient settings is well recognised in the nursing literature (Laker, Gray and Flach, 2010; Price and Baker, 2012).

Many mental health nurses repeatedly experience volatile clinical situations in different inpatient settings (Laker *et al.*, 2010; Stewart and Bowers, 2103). The health and safety of both themselves, the team and the service user(s) may be compromised as a result, if not managed successfully. In addition the therapeutic relationship may be irrevocably damaged. The Nursing and Midwifery Council (2015) confirms the nurse's duty to ensure that service users are treated appropriately, and with dignity and respect at all times, to achieve objectives. Working to minimise the potential for volatility is, therefore, a clear expectation of the nurse.

The general organisation and structure of mental health care services, the immediate clinical environment, service users themselves and clinicians can contribute to the potential for volatility, the development of aggression and the process for managing this (Cutcliffe and Riahi, 2013). Excellent communication skills and a high level of self-awareness form the basis of professional practice for mental health nurses. Competent use of specific knowledge and skills is employed to assess and manage volatile clinical situations. A positive attitude underpins practice. Rogers' (1961) principles of demonstrating congruence, unconditional positive regard and empathic understanding (see Chapter 3) should guide practice.

This chapter will consider the nature of de-escalation set in the context of clinical risk assessment and management, particularly in the context of hospital care. Ultimately the remit of this chapter is to identify the specific knowledge and skills that student nurses can consider using to de-escalate volatile situations, and offer clinical scenarios to practise these.

Learning objectives

After reading this chapter, you will:

- understand the significance of de-escalation in nursing practice
- recognise the skills of de-escalation
- know the importance of risk assessment and management
- appreciate the importance of maintaining a therapeutic relationship with the service user.

Theoretical basis

Knowing and understanding the individual service user and the factors that contribute to volatility, and that trigger or influence verbal aggression, is important. Webb (2012) emphasises the importance of clinical evaluation to establish the likelihood of events happening. The RCN (2008) notes that the nurse must become acquainted with clinical risk assessment and management. The identification of specific risks (including what, to whom, when, where and why) is critical, along with consideration of the potential outcomes and strategies to reduce risks and learn from what happens. The risk assessment should include both expert professional opinion and actuarial tools (Sturrock, 2012).

Historical factors in prediction are important. For example, knowing that certain events or circumstances have led the service user to become verbally aggressive in the past can help predict specific risks. Armed with this knowledge, measures can be put in place to reduce the likelihood of triggers happening again where possible.

Dynamic clinical variables (the things that influence the situation now for a service user, such as mental state, levels of frustration and physical environment) can change quickly, leading to a change in the service user's ability to regulate their emotional state and causing an increase in their general arousal. Initially, it might sometimes be difficult to know what the trigger is. For the service user the increased level of arousal brought on by thoughts and feelings induces the 'fight or flight' reflex. The hypothalamus, pituitary gland and adrenal gland (known collectively as the HPA axis) work together to release adrenaline to ensure that the person is physically able to respond to the heightened arousal (Smith and Vale, 2006; Goldstein, 2010). There are physical warning signs of heightened arousal caused by the release of adrenaline, such as restlessness and pacing, and other obvious identifiers of physical arousal (increased rate of breathing and heart rate, and pupil dilation). Service users may refuse to be drawn into communication or may lack concentration.

As an example, a service user newly admitted to a ward might be unsure of what is happening to them or where they are, and may experience fear of the unknown. Another service user may be alarmed by the content of their hallucinations and become confused, angry or afraid. People in these circumstances are in volatile situations and verbal aggression as a result of fear or anger can be the next natural stage in response to these emotions and physical arousal.

Specific verbally aggressive behaviours have been identified by Stewart and Bowers (2013), and include the use of abusive language (swearing, being deliberately offensive and degrading, using sexually inappropriate language, name calling, making threats), shouting and screaming, making racist comments and overt expressions of anger. More generically they noted that being 'hostile', 'argumentative' and 'irritable' (p. 239) could also be considered verbal aggression. De-escalation skills are employed to defuse volatile situations, minimising verbal aggression and avoiding physical aggression whenever possible. As well as avoiding conflict, the aim is to maintain the service user's dignity, thinking about how to help the service user better manage the aggressive expression of anger or fear.

De-escalation is a series of interconnected verbal and non-verbal skills employed by mental health nurses when working with service users who appear to be expressing distress and potential volatility. Sometimes known as 'talking down', Stevenson and Otto (1998, cited in RCN, 2006, p. 27) note that it is often perceived as an easy, simple process, but contend that 'it is actually a complex, interactive process in which a service user is redirected towards a calmer personal space'.

The ward is a busy environment and the nurse will need to ensure they spend time with the service user in any circumstances, and certainly when they present as volatile and unpredictable (Price and Baker, 2012; Stewart and Bowers, 2013). Reducing external stimulation is also helpful (Sutton et al., 2013), meaning that moving to a quieter space is appropriate, following consultation with colleagues.

In order to engage successfully at the first point of contact, the nurse must give the service user their undivided attention. The skills of active listening are brought to the fore. First, appropriate body language is considered. The nurse must *look* approachable, being conscious of their physical presentation. For example, standing with arms crossed can suggest that the nurse isn't listening, they are 'closed', whether or not that is the intended message. There may be cultural or gender considerations of some elements of communication such as eye contact (Halter, 2014). Length of eye contact may be linked to social and professional perceptions of superiority or inferiority (Burnard and Gill, 2009). In this context eye contact perceived by the service user as too long may be considered threatening or discomfiting, or as too short, evidence of a dismissive and uninterested attitude. Similarly, the therapeutic use of touch must be used deliberately and selectively at the nurse's discretion (Gleeson and Higgins, 2009).

When verbally communicating the nurse must take their time and talk at a slow pace, use short sentences and avoid technical language. Pitch, tone and volume of voice need to be regulated (Bowers *et al.*, 2010). The *way* in which the nurse speaks with the service user is as important as what is said.

A quiet resolution to engage the service user and encourage them to keep communicating may be needed (Bowers *et al.*, 2010). Questions or statements can be repeated in certain circumstances without appearing rude or forceful, and nurses must ascertain when this is appropriate. For instance, the service user experiencing auditory hallucinations may be distracted or be thinking very quickly and not paying attention to detail, so is possibly missing aspects of the conversation

Encouragers, such as head nods, brief invitations to continue ('please tell me more'), reflection and paraphrasing can be used to manage and direct the conversation, helping communication channels to remain open. Paraphrasing demonstrates interest and ensures understanding. It can help the service user to consider what they think and feel when spoken out loud. 'Autonomy confirming interventions' (Price and Baker, 2012) empower the service user to think about problem solving, and perhaps alternative ways of expressing thoughts and emotions.

Price and Baker (2012) found that being honest and open, offering care without judgement and demonstrating empathy are critical. The nurse must appear to be calm (even when this is not the case) and approach the interaction in a non-confrontational manner, remembering that this is not about 'winning or losing'. Therapeutic engagement can continue to be useful during de-escalation both to maintain a rapport with the service user and to progress the risk assessment process (Price and Baker, 2012).

The act of sometimes just 'being with' the service user as an intentional intervention is noteworthy (Bowers *et al.*, 2010). If the service user is too distressed to talk but still wants some therapeutic contact, then 'being with' might be an option. The time could be spent quietly or the nurse could use conversational distraction, talking about unimportant things, nothing related to the seriousness of the service user's current circumstances.

Constant or special observations of the service user are sometimes initiated as a preventative measure to maintain the safety of vulnerable service users (Stewart, Bowers and Ross, 2012), including those at risk because of their perceived volatility or unpredictability. Though potentially intrusive, special observations do give nurses the opportunity to spend time and engage with the service user, while also contributing to maintaining safety and risk assessments (Mackay, Paterson and Cassells, 2005).

The following scenarios, beginning with Boxes 13.1 and 13.2, represent typical examples of the nurse in practice understanding and de-escalating volatile situations.

Box 13.1 Introducing Henry

Henry, who is 20 years old, was readmitted to the acute admissions ward two days ago. He is detained under Section 2 of the Mental Health Act for England and Wales (1983, amended 2007). Henry has been experiencing disturbing visual and auditory hallucinations, and has not been very communicative since his arrival.

Staff nurse Jenny can see Henry on the ward. She notices he seems tense, pacing around the ward and glaring angrily around him. Jenny consults with her colleagues and decides to approach Henry to ask if he is OK and to make an assessment. On approaching Henry it is clear that he is not OK at all. Jenny notes that his facial expression is tense, he is breathing quite rapidly and, when she speaks to him, he stares intently at her but refuses to speak and is clearly distracted.

Henry's level of arousal is increasing and there is a clear need for Jenny to intervene to prevent an escalation of the potentially volatile situation. Jenny's aims are to diffuse the situation while maintaining Henry's dignity and safety, and that of those around him, to encourage Henry to communicate and start to develop a rapport with him. She also aims to make observations to inform the dynamic risk assessment process.

Jenny asks Henry if he would like to come and talk with her in a more private environment, ensuring that she is not alone but knowing that reducing external stimulation is often useful. Jenny knows that it is important to appear to remain calm and in control of herself. She ensures that the tone and volume of her speech are even and low. She thinks about her body language, with an open posture and making sure she physically attends to Henry, clearly giving him time and space to think.

Jenny: Hi Henry, my name is Jenny, I'm one of the staff nurses on the ward. Thanks for coming to talk with me. You seem a bit tense. Is everything OK with you? [*Jenny is being respectful and polite. She gives Henry time to think, addressing him by name*]

Henry: Well, no actually *nothing* is OK, *this* is not OK, but no one bothered asking me!' [*Henry's breathing rate is increasing and he is staring at Jenny, leaning forward towards her, his face and his body are tense. He is talking quite loudly*]

Jenny: That doesn't sound very good. Perhaps you and I could talk now? [*Jenny is using an empathic response. She is showing interest and trying to engage Henry. She is also aware of her own body language and positioning as well as that of Henry*]

Henry: What good would that do? You're just like all the rest! Don't care about me! [*Henry is becoming more animated. Jenny has to let him know that she is interested in him, and his thoughts and feelings. She decides to ask him about how he's feeling rather than argue that she does care about him*]

Jenny: It might help to talk about how you're feeling Henry. It sounds like you're not feeling good. [*Jenny is offering understanding of, or an interest in, understanding Henry's emotions*]

Henry: Of course I'm not feeling good! [*Henry's face looks angry and tense, and he is staring at Jenny*]

Jenny: OK. How about if you tell me you why you've come here. Would that be a good place to start? [*Jenny is trying to focus Henry on the here and now and to avoid confrontation. Jenny knows why Henry is here but his own perception of his experience is all important. She is persevering, having decided that it's OK to do so, and that it probably won't irritate Henry any further*]

Henry: I don't know, but I expect you're going to tell me are you, Miss Know All? [*Jenny must be honest as Henry has asked a direct question about himself and his care. Dishonesty now might damage the future therapeutic relationship. She decides to encourage Henry to talk about what happened to him when he was admitted. She does not respond to the derogatory name calling*]

Jenny: Henry, do you remember coming here yesterday? [*This must be delivered in a non-threatening manner. It is simply a question*]

Henry: Yes. So what? [*Jenny wants to help Henry explore his understanding of what happened, as she thinks he might be confused. She must be careful not to undermine or contradict this*]

Jenny: Well when you came in I think you were very distressed. [*This is a statement not a question, it is honest*]

Henry: Yes, and ...?

Jenny: OK, can you remember why you were distressed? [*Jenny gives Henry the space to think about this*]

Henry: I dunno, I just got chucked in a car and then dragged into this dump.

Jenny: That must have been very difficult for you, Henry. [*Jenny offers Henry empathy, acknowledging his experiences and he starts to relax physically*]

Henry: Of course it was! [*Jenny must be careful not to reignite Henry's agitation*]

Jenny: Perhaps you can tell me more about it. It might help.

The word 'help' is useful as it could indicate that either Henry could be helped to articulate his feelings or understand the situation better or that *he* could help Jenny understand. Jenny will listen to Henry, will not correct him, and will not be confrontational or judgemental. She is aware of the impact that what she says or does might have on Henry, but she must be open and honest. Jenny will continue to encourage Henry to communicate with her using the verbal and non-verbal skills of active listening in order to defuse the volatile situation.

Jenny has been talking with Henry (not *to* him or *at* him) in a calm, non-threatening manner, and she has demonstrated empathy and treated him with respect. Having to think quickly and be flexible, Jenny has encouraged Henry to take the lead, helping to empower him.

From this interaction Jenny has noted that Henry does not understand why he is here but he can remember coming here. She can see that Henry is able to articulate himself and she has started to form a therapeutic relationship with him. Engaging with Henry at an early stage seems to have defused the situation. Jenny has achieved the aims she set.

Box 13.2 Introducing Cora

Cora is 34 years old and has been diagnosed with schizo-affective disorder. She has been admitted to the ward several times over the past ten years. When living at home, Cora regularly avoids interaction with the community mental health team. Her mental state deteriorates quickly when she refuses to take medication regularly. Cora has been on the ward for a couple of weeks.

During previous admissions when Cora's mood was low she experienced certain auditory hallucinations (i.e. one voice in particular) that triggered self-harming behaviours including Cora cutting herself on her arms. Warning signs for this include becoming distracted and withdrawn, and Cora isolating herself on the ward.

Cora is sitting on the ward. She has moved her chair to face the wall, is rocking backwards and forwards, and has wrapped her arms around herself in a protective manner. The ward is loud, with a lot of activity.

Staff nurse Sheila consults with her colleagues and decides to approach Cora and ask her how she is feeling. Cora is breathing heavily, her eyes are wide open, with dilated pupils, and she looks scared. Cora takes a minute to respond to Sheila and is prompted to do so when Sheila keeps talking, kneels at her side and touches her very lightly on the shoulder.

Sheila's aims are to assess the volatility of the situation and defuse it, and to maintain Cora's dignity and safety and that of those around her. She also aims to help Cora to communicate and develop a rapport, as well as to continue observations and conduct a risk assessment.

Sheila asks Cora if she would like to come with her to a more private environment, ensuring she is not alone and that members of the team know where she is. Cora is wary but follows Sheila to a side room. Sheila is aware of her own body language, adopts an open position and takes her time to engage verbally with Cora.

> *Sheila:* Thanks for coming to speak with me Cora. My name's Sheila, I'm one of the staff nurses here on the ward. [*Cora does not reply or make eye contact, and keeps looking down at her hands in her lap. Sheila has made a polite and respectful introduction. There is a deliberate moment of silence as Sheila thinks that Cora might need time to think. Sheila uses Cora's name to indicate that she is engaging with her only. Sheila notes Cora's apparent physical withdrawal*]
>
> *Sheila:* You looked a bit stressed. I wondered how are you feeling Cora?
> [*Cora does not reply and does not change her position*]
>
> *Sheila:* We're a bit concerned about you Cora, and would like to help. [*Sheila is using a slow, deliberate pace and an even tone of voice, allowing the use of silence as needed. She has used Cora's name to help Cora know she is talking with her, trying to focus her on the here and now, having stated the purpose of the conversation. Sheila persists in trying to help Cora to communicate. Sheila decides to address Cora in a slightly louder voice; she leans forward to try to catch Cora's eye*]
>
> *Sheila:* Cora, can you hear me?
>
> *Cora:* [*looks up, surprised*] YES! [*Cora is clearly very distressed and looks as if she is about to cry*]
>
> *Sheila:* Cora, try to look at me please. [*Cora looks at Sheila, who continues slowly and deliberately in a calm voice. This is not confrontational but trying to focus the service user on this moment in time*]
>
> *Sheila:* Cora, when you look at me can you hear me speaking to you clearly?
> [*Cora nods*]
>
> *Sheila:* Are you hearing other voices at the moment?
>
> *Cora:* [*looks puzzled*] I don't know. [*Sheila has to reword her question to help Cora understand what she means. Cora may be distracted, she might not have understood the question or she might not have heard it*]
>
> *Sheila:* Can you hear anyone else speaking at the same time as me? [*This question is spoken in an even, non-judgemental manner*]
>
> [*Cora shakes her head*]
>
> *Sheila:* I can see that this is very difficult for you Cora. [*Sheila is demonstrating empathy*]

> Cora: [nods] I don't want to talk now. [*Sheila has to change direction; it is clear that Cora does not want to talk at this moment and Sheila will need to revisit this another time*]
>
> Sheila: Perhaps we could just sit together here quietly. [*Sheila offers Cora an alternative to talking about how she is feeling. Cora does not respond initially, so after a few moments' silence, Sheila rewords the statement into a question*]
>
> Sheila: OK, shall we just sit together for a bit?
>
> Cora: OK. [*Cora comes to sit closer to Sheila*]

Sheila has demonstrated empathy with Cora. She has engaged in active listening, and tried to start and maintain a dialogue with Cora. Sheila offered Cora a number of opportunities to start to communicate verbally, but Cora is not ready and/or does not want to, and Sheila has respected this. Sheila has picked up that, at the moment, Cora is not hearing voices, but could not determine the precise cause of Cora's deep distress and fear at this time. Cora is not able to articulate herself at the moment, but she clearly needs support.

Offering Cora the time to sit and 'be with' is as important as talking. Sheila feels comfortable with the silence and Cora asking to hold her hand indicates that Cora appreciates this interaction. Sheila and Cora have started to build a rapport.

With regard to her aims, Sheila has been able to defuse the volatility, but has not been able to find the cause of Cora's distress. Sheila has maintained Cora's dignity and safety, and that of those around her. Although Sheila has not helped Cora to verbalise what she is feeling, she has ascertained that Cora does want to engage therapeutically.

Box 13.3 summarises some of the key learning points of this chapter.

Box 13.3 Important points to consider when de-escalating volatile situations

1. Early Intervention through observation
2. Engagement and active listening
3. Flexibility/creativity
4. Be non-confrontational and non-judgemental
5. Set aims
6. Develop and maintain rapport
7. Link to risk assessment

Conclusion

This chapter started with the observation that, on occasion, people using mental health services may become volatile and unpredictable. Mental health nurses must be aware of potential risks when working with vulnerable clients, and risk assessment and management strategies must be part of the care plan. Verbal de-escalation skills are essential for maintaining safety and ensuring respect and dignity, and throughout the therapeutic relationship can be developed and maintained.

Activities

Activity 1

Recall a volatile clinical situation that you have been involved in or witnessed, perhaps like the ones with Henry or Cora. Reflecting on the situation now, and thinking about what you noticed at the time, answer the following questions.

1. What triggers were there to cause the situation, and can you identify others now? Write down the triggers you noted at the time and any you can think of now, on reflection.
2. What warning signs were there, and what other signs can you think of now? Write down the warning signs you noted at the time and any you can think of now, on reflection.
3. Identify and note down specific skills that were used to help diffuse the situation.
4. What else (if anything) do you think could have been done, or what could have been done differently?

Activity 2

When discussing your learning needs with your mentor on placement, specify one outcome to gain a better understanding of the practice of the theory of risk assessment and management applied to verbal aggression and volatility. Take time to look through the clinical risk assessment and management plans for service users who may demonstrate verbal and/or physical aggression. Pay special attention to the risk assessment tools used and the individual management plans that are in place to minimise risk and how nurses refer to this in practice. Throughout your placement, record your developing understanding of how theory is applied to practice through regular reflections.

Think carefully about your own role as a student nurse in contributing to the assessment and plan. Remember to ask questions if you aren't sure what you should do and always feed back your experiences to your mentor/the nurse in charge.

At the end of your placement, bring your reflections to the final meeting with your mentor to discuss your experiences and what you have learned. You can then identify whether you have met the aim of gaining a better understanding of the practice of clinical risk assessment and management in this area.

Suggested reading

Howatson-Jones, L. (2010) *Reflective Practice in Nursing*. Exeter: Learning Matters Ltd.

This book introduces reflection in a clear and practical way, and shows how it can support nurses in practice.

Bowers, L., Brennan, G., Winship, G. and Theodoridou, C. (2009) *Talking with Acutely Psychotic People. Communication Skills for Nurses and Others Spending Time with People Who are Very Mentally Ill*. London: City University.

This publication draws on the practice of expert nurses, who share their methods through a series of interviews.

References

Bowers, L., Brennan, G., Winship, G. and Theodoridou, C. (2010) How expert nurses communicate with acutely psychotic patients. *Mental Health Practice*, 13, 24–26.

Burnard, P. and Gill, P. (2009) *Culture, Communication and Nursing*, 2nd edition. Harlow: Pearson Education Limited.

Cutcliffe, J.R. and Riahi, S. (2013) Systemic perspective of violence and aggression in mental health. *International Journal of Mental Health Nursing*, 22, 568–578.

Department of Health (2011) *No Health Without Mental Health*. London: Department of Health.

Department of Health (2014) *Positive and Proactive Care: Reducing the Need for Physical Interventions*. London: Department of Health.

Department of Health, Social Services and Public Safety (2007) *Mental Health and Wellbeing*. Belfast: Department of Health.

Gleeson, A. and Higgins, M. (2009) Touch in mental health nursing. An exploratory study of nurses views and perceptions. *Journal of Psychiatric and Mental Health Nursing*, 16, 385–389.

Goldstein, D.S. (2010) Adrenal responses to stress. *Cellular and Molecular Neurobiology*, 30, 1433–1440.

Halter, M. (ed.) (2014) *Varcolis' Foundations of Psychiatric Mental Health Nursing. A Clinical Approach*, 7th edn. St Louis, MO: Saunders.

Health and Safety Executive (1974) *The Health and Safety at Work Act*. London: Department for Work and Pensions.

Laker, C., Gray, R. and Flach, C. (2010) Case study evaluating the impact of de-escalation and physical intervention training. *Journal of Psychiatric and Mental Health Nursing*, 17, 222–228.

Mackay, I., Paterson, B. and Cassells, C. (2005) Constant or special observations of inpatients presenting a risk of aggression or violence: nurses' perceptions of the rules of engagement. *Journal of Psychiatric and Mental Health Nursing*, 12, 464–471.

National Institute for Health and Clinical Excellence (2015). *Violence and Aggression: Short-term management in mental health, health and community settings* [NG10]. London: National Institute for Clinical Excellence.

Nursing and Midwifery Council (2015) *The Code: professional standards for practice and behavior for nurses and midwives*. London: Nursing and Midwifery Council.

Price, O. and Baker, J. (2012) Key components of de-escalation techniques: a thematic synthesis. *International Journal of Mental Health Nursing*, 21, 310–319.

Rogers, C.R. (1961) *On Becoming a Person. A Therapist's View of Psychotherapy.* New York: Houghton Mifflin Company.

Royal College of Nursing (2006) *Clinical Practice Guidelines: National Institute for Health and Clinical Excellence (2005) Violence: The Short-term Management of Disturbed/Violent Behaviour in In-patient Psychiatric Settings and Emergency Departments.* London: Royal College of Nursing.

Royal College of Nursing (2008) *Work-related Violence: An RCN Tool to Manage Risk and Promote Safer Working Practices in Health Care.* London: Royal College of Nursing.

Scottish Government (2012) *Mental Health Strategy 2012–2015.* Glasgow: Scottish Government.

Smith, S.M. and Vale, W.W. (2006) The role of the hypothalamic pituitary adrenal axis in neuroendocrine responses to stress. *Dialogues in Clinical Neuroscience*, 8, 383–395.

Stewart, D. and Bowers, L (2013) Inpatient verbal aggression: content, targets and patient characteristics. *Journal of Psychiatric and Mental Health Nursing*, 20, 236–243.

Stewart, D., Bowers, L. and Ross, J. (2012) Managing risk and conflict behaviours in acute psychiatry: the dual role of constant special observation. *Journal of Advanced Nursing*, 68, 1340–1348.

Sturrock, A. (2012) Assessing the risk of aggression and violence among service users. *Mental Health Practice*, 15, 26–29.

Sutton, D., Wilson, M., Van Kessle, K. and Vanderpyl, J. (2013) Optimizing arousal to manage aggression: a pilot study of sensory modulation. *International Journal of Mental Health Nursing*, 22, 500–511.

Webb, L. (2012) Tools for the job: why relying on risk assessment tools is still a risky business. *Journal of Psychiatric and Mental Health Nursing*, 19, 132–139.

Welsh Government (2010) *Mental Health (Wales) Measure.* Cardiff: Welsh Government.

Part 3
Working with families and groups

14

Working systemically with families in mind

Billy Hardy

Introduction

This chapter casts its net into the field of systemic therapies sometimes referred to as family therapies. This casting will include a review of ideas and practices that have influenced this field of therapy, including narrative approaches and both constructivist and social constructionist frameworks. A brief overview is offered, by way of orienting the reader, highlighting some of the key exponents and ideas that have contributed to this evolving field.

McGoldrick, Gerson and Petry (2008) write about the family life cycle, in a way that helps us to understand where and how to locate therapy techniques in face-to-face practice. This chapter also draws on aspects of the interactional communication theory of Watzlawick, Weakland and Fisch (1974), and on systemic thinking and narrative therapies (Durrant, 1989; White, 2007). It also focuses on the techniques associated with problem formation, definition and change (Lipchik, 2002; de Shazer et al., 2007), and on the technique of externalisation or external conversations.

Learning objectives

After reading this chapter, you will:

- understand how to use genograms to enhance understanding of the relational context of problems
- be able to make distinctions between problem formation, identification and resolution

- know how key contextual factors can inhibit and enhance therapeutic outcomes with service users, and how to create choice and the potential for change
- appreciate how therapists can position themselves as collaborators in service user change
- understand and be able to utilise the technique of externalisation.

Theoretical basis

Systemic family therapy has moved on from its early roots. These lie in the Milan School, the work of Pallazolli *et al.* (1978) and (in the UK) in the pioneering contribution of the Family Institute Cardiff (Dowling *et al.*, 1982; Jones, 1993) and the Tavistock London (Strickland-Clark, Campbell and Dallos, 2000). Other important influences have come from the Palo Alto group, interactional communication theorists such as Watzlawick *et al.* (1974), the schizophrenia family studies from the early 1990s (Leff, 2000) and the London depression trial (Leff *et al.*, 2000).

More recently, the latter part of the twentieth century witnessed the evolution of the so-called post-modernist therapies. This has seen an increase in approaches such as solution focused (de Shazer *et al.*, 2007) and narrative (Roth and Epston, 1996; White, 2007) therapies, through to the more collaborative, language system oriented, approaches of Andersen and Goolishian (1988). Other newer developments include the social constructionist thinking of McNamee and Gergen (1992). The push towards a more evidence-based approach to therapy has seen all therapeutic approaches coming under greater scrutiny from both inside and outside the world of practice (Stratton, 2011). The work of Lask and Waugh (2013) in eating disorders provided a platform for influencing and developing clinical practice, while a generation of practitioners has been influenced by systemic approaches to working with mental illnesses such as schizophrenia (Burbach, 2013). Couples therapy approaches now developing across the UK are building on the work of Jones and Asen (2000), and the childhood depression studies of Campbell *et al.* (2003) provide a useful foundation for continued work in this field. Strategic and policy initiatives have also begun to shape the way interventions are designed and delivered. For example, a current competencies framework for systemic therapies has highlighted a variety of skills in which practitioners can usefully engage (Pilling, Roth and Stratton, 2008). Initiatives by the NHS in England, such as the Improving Access to Psychological Therapies programme, have seen a potential reshaping and demand for specific therapeutic skills, including from mental health nurses.

Against this background, the techniques in this chapter are drawn from some of the competencies outlined by Pilling *et al.* (2008). These highlight techniques to promote change for individuals, couples and families, to help them work towards problem resolution and to aid them in the process of externalising problems.

Mapping the relational context of the problem

Mapping the relational context is a technique or a way of practice that is useful at any stage of problem formation. This may be worked through by using a genogram (McGoldrick *et al.*, 2008) or a family map. Many practitioners and students will be familiar with the family tree as a way of collecting information about the service user's relationships.

Genograms can provide a three-generational snapshot of the context of the service user, and this can be important in problem formation and eventual resolution. They can include important relationships, ages, deaths, births and events such as leaving home. They also help to locate the problem in a particular set of relationships involving the family, kinship group or others. They can illuminate important relationships with friends, pets and with the interests of the service user. Genograms can lead to explorations of stories, myths and ways of living that form part of the culture of the family. Attachments past, present and future may emerge, as well as those that have become fractured, broken or disconnected by separation, divorce, physical and mental illness, and migration in and out of the family (Dallos and Draper, 2015).

Assessment and formulation are key to mapping the system. As Pilling *et al.* (2008) have suggested, this refers to mapping the relational context of the problem. Family structure, life cycle, patterns of living, life events, and family functioning and relational patterns can be worked out through this technique. For some service users and families a journey through the maze of referral pathways is often guided by whatever problem definition is offered by way of diagnosis, behavioural description or relationship difficulty. However, by the time the referred service user moves through the health system, the problem can be seen as having taken on a life of its own. Therefore, it is important to have a clear definition from the service user of how they see the problem now, what it means and its context in relation to the service user's life.

Some of the questions discussed below may be useful starting points for practitioners and students.

When did this become a problem?

If a family is present, ask family members as well if possible.

- Who noticed it first? *This helps provide a timeline and can be asked of all family members.*
- In relation to the problem, who has been most helpful so far?
- What was life like before the problem was around? *This attempts to get a picture from the past, including past relationships and the context.*
- Who noticed the problem most once it became apparent? *This will help in identifying who is closest to being a key helper or organiser.*

- When is the problem likely to cause most harm or irritation?
- Do you have a specific name or definition of the problem? *When asking this many different definitions may emerge, and this adds a richness for exploration.*
- Who is it most a problem for: you or another member of the family? *This can elicit where the problem has had an unintended impact on another person.*
- When is the problem less noticeable?
- Who would be most pleased if the problem disappeared or got better?
- How would you know that your problem was somehow changing?
- How would those closest to you know that there is a change to you and the problem?

Introducing questions about change gives the therapeutic relationship a future orientation, and in the early connections with service users and families helps introduce the idea that change has already begun.

Box 14.1 summarises some key points from the chapter so far.

Box 14.1 Key points

- Problem formation, identification and resolution are key to understanding and connecting with service users.
- Using genograms increases the practitioner's understanding of the context.
- Mapping the relational context is a key practice and can be seen as a useful addition to assessment processes.

Externalisation of the problem

Having been purposeful and mapped the relational context of the problem, the practitioner will be able to utilise techniques within the therapeutic relationship. This technique can be used for a wide range of problems and has been utilised in a number of clinical contexts, such as eating disorders and conduct disorders, and in various adult mental health care settings, including drug and alcohol services.

Externalisation of the problem is an approach where service users are invited to objectify the problem, in a way that personifies it and sees it as 'other'. White (1989) developed this technique almost 30 years ago and it is now an established technique in the systemic field (Durrant, 1989; Duran *et al.*, 2000; Dykes and Neville, 2000; Bello, 2011). One of the more important conceptual frames for this practice is encapsulated in the idea that it is not the person, or his or her relationship, that is the problem: it is the problem itself that is 'the problem' (White, 1989). Problems can often seem toxic, and this technique can have a dissolving effect on the nature of blame in relationships. Separating the problem from the person can make it possible for the therapist and the service user to search for unique outcomes (Parry and Doan, 1994), and provide a context for shared and collaborative action.

In order to apply the technique of externalising, the problem needs to be understood in terms of who and what influences the service user's perception of the problem. Durrant (1989) has suggested that it is not simply a clever reframe or renaming of a problem, but an invitation to a service user or family to find new ways of living with the problem. This approach is illustrated below, beginning with Box 14.2, which introduces Peter.

Box 14.2 Introducing Peter and his family

Peter is a nine-year-old boy who has been experiencing temper outbursts. His mother, father and schoolteacher are all concerned with this presenting behaviour. Following careful mapping of the relational context the therapist works with the family and their son. The genogram for Peter and his family looks like this:

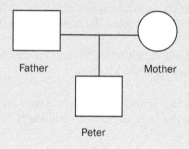

Therapist: Have you ever heard of my special traps for catching tempers when they come to visit you and your mum and dad?

Peter: No. What's that about?

Therapist: Sometimes, when boys like you have tempers that seem to just happen and explode for no reason, we can trap the temper and begin to take charge of it rather than it being in charge when it arrives. This takes a bit of time but with training some other boys have been very successful in training it.

The therapist may have some artefacts such as drawings from previous service users or examples of traps. This will help in creating a connection with the young person.

Peter: How do we do that? How do you get one?

Therapist: Well, we need a couple of things to make this work. First, we need the help of your mum and dad, and anyone else who is important in your home life. Is that OK?

Parental figures are important in the success of such an intervention.

> *Peter:* Yes, that would be great.
> *Therapist:* We also need to have someone who can verify the trap and make the special licence for you to own it, and that's me. So I can work with you, build your special trap that fits in your home and you can also have a small pocket version you can take to school. Most boys have these two special parts. What do you think? ... It's a bit like magic, but it is hard work.

Peter has had problems in school, so a mini trap that can fit in his pocket can help in other contexts. His teacher is informed and is keen to collaborate.

> *Peter:* [*excited to get started*] What do we do then?
> *Therapist:* [*talks with the parents*] Are you both able to help Peter and me?
> *Parents:* Of course. What do we need to do?
> *Therapist:* First, we need to find out when and where it happens most. Peter, can you tell me about it, can you draw it for example? You can use my iPad to do that ... [*Peter likes the idea of using the iPad*]

Peter makes a drawing and is helped by his dad on this occasion. This is part of the mapping of the influence of the problem.

> *Therapist:* Because this is such an individual trap and only for those special enough to have the trap, we need to build and design it ourselves.

Peter tells the therapist about the last time his temper came to visit. His mum was there in the house, and his dad was still on his way home. Usually it's before or after school, in the morning or the evening. The therapist is making this individual to Peter and mapping the relationship around the problem.

> *Therapist:* If you could give this a name, what would you call it, Peter?
> *Peter:* I think I will call it 'Horrible Horace'.
> *Therapist:* That's a pretty good name; very scary really. So when 'Horrible Horace' came to visit what was happening?

Here the therapist maps the relational context and gets a sense of the types of behaviours that surround the 'Horrible Horace' temper. Naming it helps in the process of personification and separation from the person.

Further exploration with the parents and the deconstruction of the moments before it happens all help towards understanding and connecting: who does what, says what, acts, how they respond, and the consequences. Exploring the meaning of the behaviour as 'Horrible Horace' removes the blaming talk that can build up over time. It also frees up the adults to have conversations with their child without the potential for escalation and destruction. The parents are also watching the therapist closely: not only are they witness to their son's problem definition and resolution, they are collaborative partners and allies.

Working with adults will take a different shape and format as the imaginative powers of children can generally generate many ideas, but for adults it is more of a challenge. Below we see this unfold, beginning with an introduction to Graham in Box 14.3.

Box 14.3 Introducing Graham and his family

Graham is a man who has recently split up from his partner and children.

He has two daughters aged 14 and 9. He has been drinking heavily and is currently off work on sick leave. Following careful conversation and mapping of the relational context, Graham in the second meeting says his drinking is problematic and is probably one of the areas of his life that led to the breakup of his relationships.

Here is the genogram for Graham and his family:

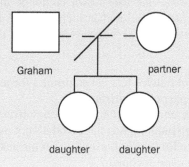

Therapist: What is your favourite drink?
Talking directly about, and with, the problem acknowledges it and offers an empathic connection.

Graham: Cider as much as possible.
Therapist: Which type of cider do you prefer: usual or flavoured?

These are questions to 'scaffold' or add context to the conversation as Graham and the therapist move forward in their talking.

Graham: Just the usual will do me.
Therapist: Have you tried the others?
Graham: No, not really. More for the younger set, I think.
Therapist: How long have you been in a relationship with cider?

Talking with the problem, and suggesting a relationship to and with it, adds to the scaffolding and to a potential personification.

> *Graham:* What do you mean 'relationship'?
> *Therapist:* How long have you and cider been together in life?
> *Graham:* I have been drinking for years, but more heavily recently.
> *Therapist:* Which brand of cider is your preference?

The therapist is mapping the influence of the problem in a non-blaming but relational frame.

> *Graham:* It's got to be Russets.
> *Therapist:* I thought so. It sounds powerful and trendy.
> *Graham:* It's the best.
> *Therapist:* Can you tell me what Russets does best for you given you are a bit of an aficionado of the stuff?

The therapist uses the service user's own language and sticks closely to his descriptions, mapping the relational influence of the problem defined, while also seeking to understand the service user's sense of himself in relation to his problem.

> *Graham:* Lately not much – just get so drunk I forget.
> *Therapist:* Is that part of the attraction?
> *Graham:* What attraction, what do you mean 'attraction'?
> *Therapist:* Well, I'm thinking you have said it's got out of hand more recently and you blame Russets [*pausing*] ... Let me ask you, if it were a person would it be man or a woman?

It is important to be explicit about preferences and description of choice.

> *Graham:* Definitely a bloke. A big bloke.
> *Therapist:* The attraction to Mr Russets is very strong, and powerful. Can I ask, was your ex-partner as attracted to Mr Russets?

Mapping the relational context, the therapist extends the invitation to talk about the drinking as a person and a dialogue emerges. It also serves to position the problem in relationship to significant others.

> *Graham:* She hated the stuff.
> *Therapist:* Was she able to see you as separate from the stuff? How about your daughters, Clare and Sara?
> *Graham:* Never really thought about it.
> *Therapist:* Have a guess what they might say.

Graham: Probably they wouldn't like it.

Therapist: You said earlier you have been drinking for a while, years before now. Twenty years? You recently split from your partner Carol and your daughters Clare and Sara, two years ago? When did you notice that you were more attracted to Mr Russets than to your family ... do you remember that?

Here the therapist is mapping the wider context. The timeframes past, present and future are important markers for dialogue and resolution. The therapist also introduces the idea of choice and responsibility.

Graham: Not really, it just crept up on me.

Therapist: Who do you prefer now, Mr Russets or your family?

Graham: I would like to see my girls.

Therapist: If Mr Russets is this big guy it sounds like he has quite a hold on you? Does he stop you from seeing your children? Do you need permission from him?

Graham: Possibly. I never thought that way about it.

Therapist: Let's say Mr Russets calls to see you, knocking on the door and you have a dilemma that evening. You have the opportunity to see your girls. What do you do? Stay in or go out with this big guy, or see your girls? What do you want most?

It is at this point that Graham has to exercise responsibility and the therapist can collaborate in building this through continued therapeutic conversations.

These extracts have highlighted two clinical contexts demonstrating the technique of externalisation. As with many therapeutic techniques, understanding and careful ethically sensitive positioning are paramount. Currently mental health nurses who are needing to expand their repertoire of practice can, through practice and attending to the stories, language and with a focus on collaborating with the potential for change, add to the richness of their practice. This expanded practice can also enrich the lives of many service users. Adopting one model of practice or following a dominant discourse of practice can deny service users access to different ways of thinking and thus potentially close down opportunities to step outside the box of self-limiting narratives about change in their lives.

Conclusion

This chapter has suggested a number of learning points. First, expand your ability in assessment with service users. Give value to joining and engaging with service users, and privilege their stories of problem description and resolution. Use genograms as a tool for talking about and contextualising problems, and to map out family and helping systems. Utilise techniques for change and problem resolution, and techniques that promote dialogue such as externalised conversations. As a mental health nurse, use yourself as a therapeutic practitioner, collaborating more with your service users and families. Share your expanding therapeutic repertoire with others and connect with other likeminded practitioners for ongoing development of thinking and practice.

Activity

Opportunities for skills development

- Join with others who are likeminded.
- Expand your reading through increasing your journal choices.
- Attend training courses and continuous professional development events, observe others working.
- Look at what's available to you, e.g. on YouTube, DVDs for training. For example, Chimamanda Adichie talks about 'The danger of the single story' at www.ted.com/talks/chimamanda_adichie_the_danger_of_a_single_story, the Association for Family Therapy and Systemic Practice has an online presence at www.aft.org.uk, as does the UK Council for Psychotherapy at www.ukcp.org.uk. Information on services and training can also be found online (for example, at The Family Institute in South Wales: http://thefamilyinstitute.southwales.ac.uk).

Suggested reading

Dallos, R. and Draper, R. (2015) *An introduction to Family Therapy*, 4th edn. Maidenhead: Open University Press.

This is an easy-to-read introduction to family therapy for practitioners from all disciplines.

Carr, A. (2012) *Family Therapy: Concepts, Process and Practice*, 3rd edn. London: Wiley.

This is a comprehensive book, combining theory, research and practical exercises.

References

Andersen, H. and Goolishian, H. (1988) Human systems as linguistic systems: preliminary and evolving ideas about the implication for clinical theory. *Family Process*, 27, 4, 371–393.

Bello, N. (2011) Narrative case study: using the client as her own witness to change. *Journal of Systemic Therapies*, 30, 2, 11–21.

Burbach, F. (2013) Developing systemically oriented secondary care mental health services. PhD thesis, University of Plymouth. Online at 2013burbach10381205phd.pdf

Campbell, D., Bianco, V., Dowling, E., Goldberg, H., McNab, S. and Pentecost, D. (2003) Family therapy for childhood depression: researching significant moments. *Journal of Family Therapy*, 25, 4, 417–435.

Dallos, R. and Draper, R. (2015) *An Introduction to Family Therapy*, 4th edn. Maidenhead: Open University Press.

de Shazer, S. and Dolan, Y. with Korman, H., Trepper, T., McCollum, E. and Berg, I.K. (2007) *More than Miracles*. London: Routledge.

Dowling, E., Cadet, B., Breunlint, D.C., Frude, N. and Seligman, P. (1982) A retrospective survey of students views on a family therapy training programme. *Journal of Family Therapy*, 4, 1, 61–72.

Duran, T.L., Cashion, L.B., Gerber, T.A. and Mendez-Ybanez, G.J. (2000) Social constructionism and eating disorders: relinquishing labels and embracing personal stories. *Journal of Systemic Therapies*, 19, 2, 23–42.

Durrant, M. (1989) The taming of temper. *Dulwich Centre Newsletter*, Autumn.

Dykes, M. and Neville, K. (2000) Taming trouble and other tales: using externalised characters in solution focused therapy. *Journal of Systemic Therapies*, 19, 2, 74–81.

Jones, E. (1993) *Family Systems Therapy: Developments in the Milan-systemic Therapies*. London: Wiley.

Jones, E. and Asen, E. (2000) *Systemic Couple Therapy and Depression*. London: Karnac.

Lask, B. and Waugh, B.R. (2013) *Eating Disorders in Childhood and Adolescence*, 4th edn. London: Routledge.

Leff, J. (2000) Family work for schizophrenia: practical application. *Acta Psychiatrica Scandinavica*, 102, Suppl. 407, 78–82.

Leff, J., Vearnals, S., Brewin, C.R., Wolff, G., Alexander, B., Asen, E., Dayson, D., Jones, E., Chisholm, D. and Everitt, B. (2000) The London depression intervention trial. *British Journal of Psychiatry*, 177, 2, 95–100.

Lipchik, E. (2002) *Beyond Technique in Solution Focused Therapy: Working with Emotions and the Therapeutic Relationship*. London: Guilford Press.

McGoldrick, M., Gerson, R. and Petry, S. (2008) *Genograms in Family Assessment*, 3rd edn. New York: W.W. Norton.

McNamee, S. and Gergen, K. (1992) *Therapy as Social Construction*. London: Sage.

Pallazolli, M.S., Boscolo, L., Cecchin, G. and Prata, G. (1978) *Paradox and Counter Paradox*. New York: Aranson.

Parry, A. and Doan, R. (1994) *Story Re-visions Narrative Therapy in the Postmodern World*. London: Guilford Press.

Pilling, S., Roth, A.D. and Stratton, P. (2008) *The Competencies Required to Deliver Effective Systemic Therapies*. London: UCL.

Roth, S. and Epston, D. (1996) Consulting the problem about problematic the relationship: an exercise for experiencing a relationship with an externalised other, in Hoyt, M.F. (ed.) *Constructive Therapies*, Vol. 2 (pp.148–162). London: Guilford Press.

Stratton, P. (2011) *The Evidence Base for Systemic Family and Couples Therapy*. Warrington: Association for Family Therapy.

Strickland-Clark, L., Campbell, D. and Dallos, R. (2000) Children's and adolescents' views on family therapy. *Journal of Family Therapy*, 22, 3, 324–341.

Watzlawick, P., Weakland, J. and Fisch, R. (1974) *Change: Principles of Problem Formation and Resolution*. New York: W.W. Norton.

White, M. (1989) The externalising of the problem. *Dulwich Centre Newsletter*, summer, special edition.

White, M. (2007) *Maps of Narrative Practice*. New York: W.W. Norton.

15

Working with groups

Alex Nute

Introduction

We live out our lives though our interactions in groups. It can be observed that human society emerges from the activity that takes place within and between interweaving groups, diverse in culture and purpose. Broad identification with a particular religion or nationality, occupation or activity can define the behaviours of group members, while inclusion in other types of group can occur through health or social status. It is important therefore to establish what the intended difference would therefore be of a therapeutic group.

Nurses, among other professions, have developed expertise in the group approach that is founded on the application of core skills such as communication and the therapeutic relationship. This chapter provides insight into the theory and practice of group work to guide the nurse towards facilitation of effective recovery-focused group practice. A review of therapeutic and supportive formats will be presented to introduce the basic processes associated with this approach, followed by a discussion of inclusive group facilitation styles. The subsequent examination of the group process forms a practical guide to undertaking facilitation roles through each stage of group activity, complemented by action points that focus on the needs of those new to group facilitation. Readers are also referred to Chapter 7 for a further discussion of, and exercises in, group working.

Learning objectives

After reading this chapter, you will:

- be able to apply a recovery philosophy to therapeutic groups
- know how to plan and organise group activity

- have confidence in practising the roles of the group facilitator
- be able to help facilitate a structured group process
- have skills in evaluating and recording the outcomes of group work.

The therapeutic group

In mental health, therapeutic groups provide an opportunity for people to rehearse aspects of their functioning in situations that closely resemble their normal social groups or setting. The group provides a 'sandbox' for participants to observe constructed social activity, offering opportunities to gain practical knowledge around communication and interaction. The group space offers permission to address alternative ways of being and behaving, guiding positive change that arises from within the culture. Finlay (1993) notes that groups allow us to monitor perceptions of the effect we have on others, and so resolve our expectations of their receptiveness and responses. This learning about social activity and testing of interpersonal skills, ideas and behaviours can occur in a safe and supportive environment.

Modern group theory draws from the empowerment ideals of the post-war therapeutic community movement, building new perspectives on therapy, mutuality and growth. These values are recycled in recovery manifestos such as the (Sainsbury) Centre for Mental Health's methodology for organisational change and statement of principles (Shepherd, Boardman and Burns, 2008; Shepherd, Boardman and Slade, 2008), which stress the importance of health care professionals being 'on tap not on top'. We are tasked therefore to challenge established hierarchies and change the nature of our interactions to redefine service user involvement, and this approach finds its practical expression in the *co-production* and *facilitation* of the therapeutic group.

Types of group

Literature describing a considerable diversity of group approaches can be drawn from across the humanities. In mental health care, approaches can be classified along a spectrum of activity-based and therapeutic styles, with considerable overlap evident in their task-specific, supportive and psychotherapeutic focus.

Structured groups are content focused, and aim to help participants develop new skills and knowledge. Examples include interactive psychoeducation groups that build understanding and acceptance, or groups that build self-management skills through learning cognitive-behavioural approaches to anxiety. Reality orientation and reminiscence groups are further variations that apply a validatory model for the cognitively impaired person, often using props such as music, images and objects.

Unstructured groups have a more heterogeneous membership, and tend towards an analytic focus on interpersonal experiences as antecedent to change.

Examples include psychoanalytic and psychodynamic groups, holding similar objectives to individual psychotherapy to which they may be a useful adjunct (Frisch and Frisch, 2011). Luffman (2009) cautions against undertaking such exploratory group approaches where participants have complex histories of maladaptive relationships, and there are concerns around trust and self-harm.

Supportive groups such as self-help, peer support and social-recreational forms provide a facility for a generally homogenous membership to seek empowerment through a sense of community and mutual aid. Shared experience is a key component, a jumping-off point to actively explore group and individual understanding, providing safety and inspiring change.

Types can be further divided between *open* groups featuring a fluid membership derived from individual need, and *closed* groups, which tend to have a fixed membership and term (as discussed in Chapter 7). Some groups seek to achieve specific tasks such as employment support/shared experience or pre-discharge preparation groups, where mutual learning can grow from the sharing of individual achievements.

Dilallo and Padmore (2013) and Croom (2009) advise that specialist knowledge of developmental stages and communication is required to pursue group approaches with young people. Facilitators particularly invest in building trusting relationships (including with parents/guardians), self-esteem and resilience to construct a nurturing social arena; for adolescent provision this moves towards an understanding of their functioning in more mature relationships to build positive self-identity, exploring the projection of 'fears, fantasies, conflicts and feelings' (Croom, 2009, p. 333).

Group process

Groups thrive or founder according to their success in constructing a sense of identity and belonging, called *cohesion*. Cohesion occurs where 'norms' of behaviour and relationships evolve through the life cycle of the group, becoming understood and internalised by participants as a prerequisite to meaningful progression. Models describing this group process tend to follow a familiar theoretical structure, as follows.

- **Orientation phase:** participants establish respective identities, begin to explore the potential of the group and agree initial rules of conduct.

- **Action phase:** characterised by sharing and experimentation. 'Norms' are accepted, though change can be both positive and transgressive; individual roles and communication vary from supportive to cathartic as the group becomes increasingly self-regulating. The possibility of positive change is accepted and actualised.

- **Termination phase:** outcomes are reviewed against the stated aims. Change is recognised and celebrated.

Progression through these phases is predicated on the *constraints* under which the group operates. These can include practical concerns such as the size and characteristics of the group or the environment in which it meets. Group dynamics may also be explored. Effective group facilitation involves the recognition of these elements and their favourable organisation for the achievement of the group's objectives.

Facilitating therapeutic groups

Planning and preparing

Finlay (1993) provides a useful sequence of actions for planning groups, as follows.

1. **Decide on type:** this will be dictated by the constraints of the hosting service and those of the target population; decisions may have been taken about the overall objective before delegation to a clinician to facilitate. Variables concerning facilitation style, specific approaches and availability of resources should however be clarified by the facilitator.

2. **Define aims:** this must provide clarity around the core work of the group, though participants will also have individual goals that will need to be accommodated. Flexibility can be an asset here, inclusive of parameters such as number and length of sessions or the intended outcomes.

3. **'Sell' the group:** how will the group meet demand? Why should the organisation and the participants commit resources to it? Producing a paper outlining the process and evaluation strategy will help consolidate your plans and keep everyone informed of the group's purpose; this should then help with the creation of information leaflets to enable service users to decide if they wish to join the group.

4. **Set membership:** Remocker and Storch (1990) advise a review of intended activity when selecting the size of the group, including the relationship to available resources of environment, staffing and commitment. Where options are available, it is important to be considerate of the interpersonal nature of the group when setting inclusion criteria: participants can be selected only through judgements of their potential to contribute positively to mutual learning and growth.

5. **Prepare group:** group members must (in most instances) be capable of providing informed consent, including understanding any potentially negative outcomes and accepting participant confidentiality. An initial 'contracting' of what behaviour or rules are acceptable in the group helps participants know what to expect.

6. **Plan sessions:** the structure of each session should mirror that of the overall group process, so is divided into the three fundamental phases outlined below. Session length is dictated by the abilities of group participants to concentrate and stay on task.

    a) *Orientation phase:* participants welcome and acknowledge one another before being brought to a review of the group's aims and objectives, progression and agenda for the session. Personal updates and reviews of homework (where applicable) are presented; early introduction of some form of whole-group activity (alternatively games or physical activities) can have positive effects on engagement with subsequent phases.

    b) *Action phase:* in early stages of the group this will include further work on orientation to expectations and norms through the development of a participant contract. As the group progresses, the activity here becomes directed to the achievement of the planned outcomes.

    c) *Termination phase*: the group winds down with reflection on activity and affirmation of the participants' contribution.

-   Further consideration should be given to the post-group reflection of the facilitator(s), including recording events and achievements. The three-stage model is otherwise flexible to meet the needs of different approaches; social or support groups may include a 'business' element before the action phase, or allow space for social activity that will enhance engagement with the therapeutic process – a brief 'break' between such elements will maintain a boundaried focus to the group's work.

Additional practical variables include venue accessibility and the use of space and seating arrangements, breakout rooms, lighting and availability of resources, and identification of the most convenient day and time for participants to meet.

Group facilitation

A key principle of recovery practice is to work with optimism (Shepherd, Boardman and Slade, 2008); this attribute defines the group facilitation style.

A participative or democratic style of leadership (Lewin, Lippitt and White, 1939) was found to be effective in offering guidance and encouraging input from members, suggesting that group involvement in decision-making processes leads to greater engagement, motivation and creativity. For recovery-focused services the alternative conception of 'facilitation' assumes change to have an internal locus that can be located and tapped when the potential for it is acknowledged and welcomed; Foulkes (1964) conceptualises group facilitation as dynamic administration of a safe space to actualise that potential. The

recovery-focused facilitator may adopt roles in leadership, support and evaluation, but does not undertake them in isolation – she or he seeks to provide the
resources that the group requests of them at each moment, free of assumptions,
with recognition of the capacity and talents of other participants to assume
those roles themselves.

This style of co-production (Perkins *et al.*, 2012) provides an overarching
conceptual framework for therapeutic groups. Inclusion of service-user experts
as co-facilitators from the point of commissioning demonstrates commitment
to recovery principles, and enhances cohesion, collaboration and motivation.
Benefits of co-facilitation including the sharing of support, and reflection will
increase in value where that partnership includes service-user expertise, through
the implicit recognition of its value and inspiration for recovery. Co-facilitation
relies on keen awareness and management of the relationship, and careful negotiation between the parties; co-facilitators should complement one another's
styles and values, but offer something distinct that can be exploited.

Facilitators should be trained and prepared to fulfil this role, and taking part
in groups and practising reflectively are important parts of this process. Co-facilitation provides exposure to the roles and behaviours that build and maintain
group direction and momentum, such as assigning roles that move participants
out of their comfort zone; encouraging quieter members to take more active
roles, or more vocal contributors to step back and observe; encouraging free,
open dialogue rather than isolated discourse; or using silence positively as an
opportunity for reflection.

The facilitator monitors and evaluates the overall mood and behaviour of
the group, and encourages a positive focus on communication. Douglas (2000)
groups the necessary tasks into four categories of moderating 'leadership acts':
smoothing/maintaining; moving/achieving; directive/focused; and, ultimately,
surviving/enhancing the group process as a whole. Facilitators should also look
to create opportunities for other participants to perform these actions.

The group process

Tuckman (1965) reviewed literature concerning a diverse typology of small
groups, reporting on an emergent 'conceptualization of changes in group behaviour ... across all group settings, over time' (p. 386). The four-stage developmental
sequence he proposes is almost ubiquitous where group processes are described,
and is used here to structure a practical guide to facilitation.

Early group phase

Stage 1: forming
The group begins by 'jostling' to establish culture and test the acceptable interpersonal boundaries. The facilitator becomes a conductor, with participants
donating a degree of personal authority to the group through defining its ground
rules.

Facilitation tasks include provision of *social-interactional* support founded in observation of the developing group dynamic. Icebreakers and games encouraging individual contributions can be used to make some initial evaluations of group development, with seating positioned 'in the round' to mitigate the tendency for early activity to focus on the facilitator. Participants may take on undifferentiated attachments, expressed through mirroring, pairing and rescuing, which foster a sense of safety and familiarity. Subgroups may begin to form as alliances help participants gain confidence and find their voice.

Individual expectations and goals should be openly discussed alongside those effecting movement towards the group's overall aim, providing both with clarity of purpose and an evaluation mechanism; participant involvement in cocreation will help to create a culture of action. A balance can be struck between encouraging freedom of expression that is idiosyncratic and comfortable, and maintaining safety – the group dynamic energises change, but through cohesion more often than conflict at this early stage.

Cohesion is similar to the psychotherapeutic concept of 'holding', arising from setting boundaries wherein emotional growth can emerge from testing and practice. Using inclusive terms such as 'us' and 'we' strengthens the sense of connectedness and identity, building concordance with the evolving norms. A key indicator of the maturation of this stage is the creation of 'ground rules'. Douglas (2000) suggests that the areas to cover may include the following (also see Chapter 7):

• why we're here
• contributing and attending
• prohibition of violence or intimidation
• equity of opportunity
• honesty
• confidentiality
• inclusiveness
• celebrating diversity.

Box 15.1 introduces a first example of a group in action.

Box 15.1 Introducing a pre-discharge group

You have been acting as co-facilitator alongside an experienced peer support worker (PSW) for a new pre-discharge group in a secondary community recovery service. The first session has arrived at the action phase.

> *PSW:* We're all clear about why we've been invited here, and discussed our hopes and expectations and all the practical stuff, so I think we should

talk about some additional ground rules. What do you think might help us to keep on track to achieve those expectations? [*facilitators observe a silence for reflection*]

Devon: We need to listen to each other.

PSW: OK, that's a good start. Why do we need to listen to one another?

Devon: Because we need to be heard.

Rani: ... and respected.

PSW: So we're not just listening, we're being respectful of others?

Rani: Everyone has a right to opinions and feelings, you know?

Carly: It's not always easy to say what I feel ... [*another pause*]

PSW: You've made a good start right there – if we're respectful of one another it encourages us to speak with more confidence. Let's add 'treating one another with respect' to our ground rules. Does that then mean we can make a statement here as well that relates to making contributions? [*The issue of respect has now brought the discussion to participant contributions and is codified into the group contract*]

Confusion and conflict phase

Stage 2: storming

In this stage members seek to define their own identity and individuality through challenging the felt restrictions of the group's newly established structure and norms. The demands of the group task provoke an emotional response that is not necessarily negative – key tasks involve the integration of group and individual goals and perceptions.

Often the most fertile ground for change lies at the margins of established group behaviours, and even where behaviour becomes transgressive, growth can occur. Previously learned and successful strategies, such as being loud and demonstrative or oppositional, can be familiar or 'safe' ways to express anxiety. Acceptance of critical reflection and the subsequent rehearsal of alternative strategies are central to group work; the facilitator may use as much energy in preventing stagnation between participants as they identify with one another's positions as they do in resolving conflict.

Facilitators must accept that they are not *responsible* for the actions of the group, but rather a *resource* to help maintain both safety and direction. The contracted ground rules help maintain a balance is struck between dynamic tension and acceptable standards of behaviour through tentative self-regulation.

A further set of skills and approaches can be offered by the facilitator to help ameliorate problems that emerge from the group dynamic. Careful facilitation of participant reflections may be required where engagement is stifled by anxiety or monopolisation by more vocal participants, or possibly a more direct challenge where the motivation and engagement of the whole group is at risk. An offer of additional individual support can be made to refocus on the mutuality of individual contributions and the group's progression. Care needs to be taken to monitor for the emergence of any scapegoating of individual participants.

Conflict can stall the group's progress where it impacts regularly on cohesiveness, risking participants becoming introverted and unresponsive. Facilitators can consider a return to more structured formative tasks, together with a review of expectations and contracting. Where there is disruption in the group, or emotional expressions that go beyond what may be processed within the dynamic, facilitators should carefully assess whether specific additional needs or clinical concerns may underlie the behaviour and act accordingly – co-facilitation here provides opportunities to re-establish behavioural norms through role modelling, or provision of individual support outside the group itself.

The enhanced potential for facilitator development through critical peer supervision is a further strength of this approach. Facilitator confidence can be at risk in this stage, and realistic expectations must be grounded in the group's culture and identity. Box 15.2 continues the example of a group in action.

Box 15.2 Continuing the pre-discharge group

The pre-discharge group is reaching the end of the conflict stage, though some issues still need to be fully resolved.

> *Carly:* I still don't think he's getting it, I ...
> *Rani:* Well, tell him then.
> *Carly:* Let me finish will you? He's ...
> *Rani:* Say it to him, not the rest of us.
> *Carly:* Will you tell her to stop that please? I'm trying to say something important here ...
> *PSW:* Let's just park things for a moment. This feels like a good opportunity to revisit our ground rules – what do you think?
> *Carly:* They're not respecting what I have to say.
> *Rani:* That's not it at all. I just think you should have the confidence to say it to Devon. [*pause*]
> *Carly:* But you just keep interrupting me and we're supposed to take turns ... Devon – I'm trying to tell you why I'm anxious, and you're just brushing it off.
> *PSW:* OK, before we carry on, let's just take a look at what's going on here in your communication with each other. [*The group discuss their interactions with reference to group norms and objectives*]

WORKING WITH GROUPS 201

Cohesion and performance phase

Stage 3: norming

The development of cohesion cements the group's norms, fostering a new open-ness in offering and interpreting personal beliefs and goals.

The group begins to reap the rewards of the earlier work that nurtured and tested its norms. The facilitator role changes to one of *enablement* as the group finds new confidence to take responsibility for progress, and may only intermit-tently need to draw on the perceived authority to maintain established bound-aries. The facilitator makes the group dynamic explicit through summary and clarification, including recognition of achievements. The facilitator also acts as a role model for these behaviours to be adopted by the group itself.

Stage 4: performing

The group reaches an action-oriented functional stage built on acceptance and mutuality. Tasks and blockages are explored, and risks taken for growth and insight. Roles become flexible within a supportive structure.

The tasks of the group are now open to completion; challenges are greeted with enthusiasm and the norms of the group become flexible to the actualising of progress. Not all groups will successfully reach this stage or remain within it, and stagnation could occur through the loss of dynamic tension – neither scenario would mean that the group has failed, however, as it is possible that the therapeutic group that reaches this stage has met its aims and outgrown its usefulness.

Termination phase

Tuckman later amended his approach to include a further stage, Stage 5: 'adjourning' (Tuckman and Jensen, 1977), which may involve a return to the lead-ership role. Emotional attachments will have been formed that can be processed through ritual activities that acknowledge and express them.

A review of the participants' performance will celebrate their achievements and acknowledge how their newly acquired skills will be useful in their lives out-side of the group. Where the group has not achieved expectations facilitators act positively to seek new directions and goals, and attempt to mitigate negative experience to maintain hope for future success. The final facilitator role begins here with the canvassing of group evaluations.

Record keeping and evaluation

Service evaluation lies at the heart of clinical governance and is integral to the nursing process. Evaluation touches the group life cycle at numerous points to report on interactions and blockages, and the performance of facilitators. Post-group reflection on outcomes provides a feedback mechanism that monitors effi-cacy and the potential for harm, with co-facilitation (particularly co-production) adding depth and quality.

Evaluation includes overt communication with the group, and ideally is openly shared with it. Feedback should be sought on exit, whether planned or unplanned, as part of a supportive package, including on facilitator performance. Where no new members are recruited for open groups a review should be made of the rationale for and accessibility of that service. In addition to the measurement of progress, evaluation contributes to planning subsequent cycles of intervention.

Record keeping is essential for effective learning about change. Participants' individual memories can be unreliable, particularly over time; slow, steady change can be missed without effective records being constructed from the facilitator's reflections at the conclusion of each session. Group records are subject to the same regulation as clinical notes in terms of their objectivity and storage; records made in clinical notes and reports to care coordinators must respect confidentiality within limits agreed by the group and set out by professional standards and the law.

Conclusion

This chapter has shown how therapeutic groups require careful planning and preparation, and how facilitation is a collaborative process that builds group cohesion. It has suggested that conflict and challenge can be uncomfortable but are also productive of change. Facilitators may adopt many roles, depending on the needs of the group, and continuous reflection and evaluation are integral to the success of the group process.

Activity

As a way of practising some of the skills outlined in this chapter, readers may wish to work through the activity opportunities below.

- Seek experience in group contexts to develop your communication and interpersonal skills. This can include taking part in open groups in practice situations, but is not limited to clinical practice – staff support groups, academic tutorials and many other activities involving the practice of social communication can be fertile ground for learning and experimentation.
- Learn from yourself and from others: experienced nurses and other professionals can help you to gain insights into group facilitation and processes, through co-facilitation, role modelling and 'apprenticeship' in practice. Take critical feedback from other participants to contextualise your reflections and supervision experiences.
- Be aware of your own limitations and act accordingly. Psychotherapeutic approaches, for instance, may require specific training and personal experience before taking up facilitation, where established support groups will benefit from your application of core skills and values.

Suggested reading

Dilallo, J. and Padmore, J. (2013) Working with groups, in Norman, I. and Ryrie, I. (eds) *The Art and Science of Mental Health Nursing: Principles and Practice*, 3rd edn (pp.367–382). Maidenhead: Open University Press.

This is a succinct chapter that contains a series of case studies demonstrating how group work can be integrated into practice.

References

Croom, S. (2009) Groupwork with children and adolescents, in Barker, P. (ed.) *Psychiatric and Mental Health Nursing: The Craft of Caring*, 2nd edn (pp.331–337). London: Hodder Arnold.

Dilallo, J. and Padmore, J. (2013) Working with groups, in Norman, I. and Ryrie, I. (eds) *The Art and Science of Mental Health Nursing: Principles and Practice*, 3rd edn (pp.367–382). Maidenhead: Open University Press.

Douglas, T. (2000) *Basic Groupwork*, 2nd edn. London: Routledge.

Finlay, L. (1993) *Groupwork in Occupational Therapy*. London: Chapman and Hall.

Foulkes, S. (1964) *Therapeutic Group Analysis*. London: Karnac Books.

Frisch, N. and Frisch, L. (2011) *Psychiatric Mental Health Nursing*, 4th edn. New York: Delmar, Cengage Learning.

Lewin, K. Lippitt, R. and White, R. (1939) Patterns of aggressive behaviour in experimentally designed social climates. *Journal of Social Psychology*, 10, 271–299.

Luffman, P. (2009) Psychodynamic approaches to working in groups, in Barker, P. (ed.) *Psychiatric and Mental Health Nursing: The Craft of Caring*, 2nd edn (pp.345–354). London: Hodder Arnold.

Perkins, R., Repper, J., Rinaldi, M. and Brown, H. (2012) *Recovery Colleges*. London: Centre for Mental Health.

Remocker, A. and Storch, E. (1990) *Actions Speak Louder: A Handbook of Structured Group Techniques*. Edinburgh: Churchill Livingstone.

Shepherd, G., Boardman, J. and Burns, M. (2008) *Implementing Recovery: A Methodology for Organisational Change*. London: Sainsbury Centre for Mental Health.

Shepherd, G., Boardman, J. and Slade, M. (2008) *Making Recovery a Reality*. London: Sainsbury Centre for Mental Health.

Tuckman, B. (1965) Developmental sequences in small groups. *Psychological Bulletin*, 63, 6, 384–399.

Tuckman, B. and Jensen, M. (1977) Stages of small-group development revisited. *Group and Organisation Studies*, 2, 4, 419–428.

16

Family intervention in psychosis

Alicia Stringfellow

Introduction

Family intervention for psychosis offers a collaborative approach aimed at working in partnership with both service users and their carers and family members. The approach builds upon existing strengths within families, and explores solutions that enable them to effectively deal with the difficulties they may face as a result of the illness. The ultimate aim of family intervention is to promote understanding of and recovery from psychosis, and to improve the individual's social functioning and independence.

This chapter will highlight the theoretical basis for family intervention for psychosis and provide a step-by-step explanation of the therapeutic skills mental health nurses can utilise to engage and support families. Particular attention will be paid to assessment and engagement, psychoeducation and communication skills. Problem solving and relapse prevention will also be highlighted in the context of family working, and consideration given to supervision and possible barriers to effective implementation.

Learning objectives

After reading this chapter, you will be able to:

- develop an appreciation of the efficacy of family intervention for psychosis, and identify the purpose, goals and benefits of the intervention
- identify the main components of family intervention for psychosis
- apply a range of communication skills to facilitate family intervention techniques with service users and their families.

Theoretical basis

Historically, there has been a plethora of theories that have hypothesised an association between the family environment and the development of psychosis. Studies conducted by Brown, Carstairs and Topping in the 1950s investigated the outcome of service users discharged from mental health hospitals in an attempt to investigate the nature of the home environment (Brown, Carstairs and Topping, 1958). The investigation resulted in the measure of expressed emotion (EE), which refers to key aspects of interpersonal relationships, including criticism, hostility, warmth, positive comments and over-emotional involvement (Brown, Birley and Wing, 1972). The correlation between EE and relapse rates has since been accepted as a robust predictor of outcome in schizophrenia (Vaughn and Leff, 1976; Kavanagh, 1992; Bebbington and Kuipers, 1994; Scazufca and Kuipers, 1996; Kuipers, 2006). Expressed emotion has been the subject of much debate over recent years and caution is necessary as families can feel unfairly blamed by health professionals for causing or contributing to mental illness. Nonetheless, the work on EE is an influencing factor within a stress-vulnerability model of psychosis (Nuechterlain and Dawson, 1984; Zubin and Spring, 1997) and has important implications for the management of the illness. The stress-vulnerability model describes an interaction between inherent and stressful environmental factors, which can result in an increased risk of episodes of the illness. By identifying and modifying such sets of stimuli it is possible to reduce, or at least delay, relapse.

Current research suggests that psychosocial interventions for those with severe mental illness can have a great impact on relapse rates, psychotic symptoms, length of stay in hospital, affective symptoms and social functioning. A significant development in the treatment of psychosis has been a change in perception of psychological interventions such that they are now recognised as an important component of a comprehensive approach (NICE, 2009, 2014).

Carer or family burden is generally regarded as long-standing and pervasive. It includes stress, anxiety, depression, physical ill-health, restrictions in leisure and social activities, financial difficulties and an overall decrease in the quality of life as a result of caring for a family member with psychosis (Doornbos, 2002; Thornicroft et al., 2004; Kuipers and Bebbington, 2005). In addition, families struggle with the symptoms associated with the service user's illness, as well as insufficient information and resources from health care providers.

The family is viewed as a valuable and underused resource in the community, with much to offer in relation to the care, treatment and support of individuals with psychosis. Family intervention aims to increase family knowledge of the condition, and coach family members in ways to manage the symptoms and stress associated with caring for their family member. This is achieved by establishing a collaborative working relationship with all family members, including the service user themselves. A positive, non-blaming attitude on the part of the mental health nurse helps to establish a working alliance where, together, family and nurse attempt to find new ways of coping and effective solutions to problems faced within the family unit (Fadden, 1998; Raune, Kuipers and Bebbington, 2004). Educating families about the service user, illness and its treatment, management and prognosis is a key component of the intervention. Its aim is to ultimately reduce stress within the family and the impact of carer burden on close family members.

In a survey by the Schizophrenia Commission (2012), 61 per cent of respondents said that family support was the most crucial factor to facilitate recovery; however, most families are understandably ill prepared to cope with a family member with psychosis, knowing very little about the condition, symptoms, treatment and prognosis. Unhelpful and stigmatising stereotypes can often lead to feelings of isolation, withdrawal and loss.

The National Institute for Health and Care Excellence (NICE) guidelines for schizophrenia over the past decade have recommended that psychosocial treatments, in conjunction with medication, become an indispensable part of the treatment options within mental health, and should be available to all service users and their families in the effort to promote recovery. More recently the guidelines were updated (NICE, 2014) with family intervention being recommended both for those with first-episode psychosis and those with subsequent episodes; furthermore that family intervention should be offered to *all* families of those with first-episode or persistent symptoms of psychosis.

In response to rising prevalence rates of mental disorders and the associated burden of psychosis, a number of family intervention training initiatives have been developed over the past two decades, including the Thorn course (Gamble, 1997), the COPE programme (Bradshaw, Lovell and Richards, 2000; Bradshaw, Mairs and Lowndes, 2003) and Behavioural Family Therapy (Falloon, Boyd and McGill, 1984). The aim of these courses has been to provide mental health professionals with the knowledge and skills to implement and deliver family intervention and other psychosocial interventions as part of their routine clinical practice. The mental health nurse therefore is well placed to use family intervention principles to help service users with psychosis and their families.

Engagement and assessment

When working with families, the building of a therapeutic relationship with each family member is just as important as the relationship between the mental health nurse and the individual service user. Trust, respect, patience and sensitivity, as well as building a positive relationship, are all key factors for therapeutic work with families to be possible. It is important that the mental health nurse recognises how past experiences and current concerns can impact on the therapeutic relationship, and the nurse should take time to engage with families so that successful engagement can occur. The nurse must demonstrate a confident, non-judgemental, enthusiastic approach when working with family members, and convey belief in the intervention and its potential successes.

Furthermore they should be approachable, reliable and interested in the family. The nurse should demonstrate a genuine, empathic and respectful attitude, while acknowledging that the family members are a valued and important support in the recovery of their loved one. For some families this may be the first encounter with mental health services or the first time a health professional has engaged with them in this way.

As mentioned previously, a non-judgemental attitude and excellent communication skills are important when working with families. Active listening skills, such as summarising and reflecting and demonstrating unconditional positive regard and empathy, are vital to the successful engagement of family members. During the initial stages of engagement, the mental health nurse should listen to the family's past experiences. This may prove challenging at times, especially if the family's experience has been a negative one. The family may voice their dissatisfaction with services or other health professionals, or may feel anger, disappointment and frustration about the lack of help and support previously. It is important that the nurse acknowledges the family's feelings towards mental health services, allowing the expression of these in an open, supportive and non-defensive manner and, in doing so, encourage the family to move forward and focus on the support that is now available.

A crucial part of the engagement process is offering an explanation to the family about family intervention as a therapeutic approach and the benefits this can bring. The intervention should be explained in terms of its effectiveness as an evidence-based approach that is collaborative in nature and focuses on the here and now rather than the past. The involvement of everyone in the family who wants to be included should be positively encouraged, and any information given should be jargon free. The family should be informed that the focus of family intervention is on identification of early warning signs, relapse prevention and management of situations within the family, as well as the development of effective problem-solving strategies and more effective methods of communication. It is useful to give the family some written material to read in their own time, and adequate time should be given for them to process and think about the information they have been given, answering any questions they may have and helping them make an informed decision as to whether they wish to commence with the intervention.

How we do it: engagement

Consider the extracts that follow.

> *Mental health nurse:* When a family member has a health problem it changes what the person can do for themselves. These changes add to the physical and emotional demands of everyday life, and can also affect how the family copes with problems and sets goals for the future. These demands are no different when the illness is a mental health problem. Relatives can

find it difficult to understand why it is that the person has difficulty doing what they used to do. As a result it is not always obvious how to help. Family intervention can support families to develop an understanding of the illness, develop effective problem-solving strategies and enhance communication between family members.

Family member: Why is it recommended that mental health professionals work with families?

Mental health nurse: Clinical trials have shown that people with psychosis are less likely to relapse when their family has received a specific therapy called family intervention for psychosis.

Family member: Why should it help?

Mental health nurse: Family members often ask for more information about the illness, how to cope with it and what the future is likely to be. Without the knowledge and skills to manage problems associated with mental health problems families often report higher levels of personal stress. High amounts of stress can lead to mental and physical health problems in family members and contribute to the risk of relapse. It is now recommended that all families who are in close contact with a family member who has a long-term mental health problem receive the intervention.

Family member: What is involved?

Mental health nurse: There are four parts to family intervention:

1. a brief assessment of each family member's knowledge and coping so that the intervention can be tailored to their needs

2. sharing information about the condition between family members

3. coaching to improve communication between family members; this can help manage symptoms and personal stress

4. providing skills in family problem solving and goal setting.

The intervention typically takes between 9 and 15 one-hour sessions. Families are asked to practise new skills between sessions. One or two mental health professionals will work with you over this time. In the session the mental health workers will encourage you to talk to one another, practise skills and solve problems.

Assessment

The process of assessment starts once the family has agreed that family intervention may be of benefit to them. As with any assessment, it is an ongoing process throughout the time the mental health nurse is working with the family. It is important to conduct individual family member assessments to determine a baseline for each person. This helps build a therapeutic relationship with each individual family member, to define each family member's understanding of the illness, to identify individual goals of family members, to define strengths, identify areas of development and to monitor progress. Usually assessments are completed in one session with each family member, however it should be recognised that some family members may find this process difficult and upsetting, so it may be more appropriate for the assessment to be conducted over multiple sessions.

In addition to gaining general background information from each family member, the following questions can be useful during the individual assessment session.

- What is your understanding of [the service user's] disorder?
- In your experience, what has made things better?
- In your experience, what has exacerbated the situation?
- What impact does the illness have on you? How is your life affected by this?
- In your own life, what would you like to be doing more or less of?
- Who do you discuss any problems with?

Box 16.1 contains an opportunity for you to engage in a learning activity.

Box 16.1 Activity opportunity

- Think about your first meeting with the family. What should you consider in developing a therapeutic relationship and successful engagement with all family members?
- What are the practical issues to be aware of and what are the potential difficulties?
- How would you promote family intervention to the family? What key points would you explain?

Psychoeducation

A major component of family intervention is psychoeducation (see Chapter 7). This enables the service user to make sense of their experiences, to help the family understand what has been happening and to help health professionals make sense of the family and the information that may assist them in managing the mental health difficulties more effectively. It is vitally important that information conveyed to the family is relevant, appropriate, evidence based, free from jargon and in a format that the family members can understand. The information should be tailored towards the specific needs of the family, and time should be given to allow all family members to discuss any issues raised, ask questions and process the information. Caution is needed when taking information from web-based sources, but using different media to help get the message across can maintain the interest and concentration of family members.

The role of the mental health nurse is to facilitate an open discussion around the features, symptoms and treatment of the illness in order to promote understanding and empathy within the family. They should be sensitive to the emotional impact of information and spend time addressing the more sensitive issues.

Families can greatly benefit from information around what will make the situation better or worse, and what to do in a crisis. Names and contact details of health professionals involved and local services, as well as suggestions of practical ways of addressing problems and managing stressful situations, are welcomed in light of an increased understanding of why these difficulties have arisen. An open and relaxed atmosphere that is conducive to the sharing of concerns, ideas and beliefs is essential. The service user should be encouraged from the outset to share their experiences in order to aid the understanding of other family members.

It is helpful to provide families with information as soon as possible following contact with mental health services. This can help prevent the development of inaccurate views of the illness, and reduce stress levels and stigma within the family.

The process of gaining information may be painful for family members and they may display signs of denial or disbelief. This is a natural process and one that can be beneficial in coming to terms with the illness. It is important for the mental health nurse to support families through this process, while acknowledging that they do not have specific answers to questions such as 'Why us?'

Box 16.2 contains an opportunity for you to engage in a further learning activity.

Box 16.2 Activity opportunity

Conduct a search for relevant material to incorporate as part of the psychoeducation element of family work. Critically analyse the material and consider the appropriateness of its use with families. Consider the content, readability and how it may feel to be on the receiving end of such information. What are the difficult parts? How would you address these in a family session?

Communication skills

When individuals are stressed, communication can become ineffective and unhelpful. This is particularly so when a family member experiences mental health problems. Families may be aware that their communication is not working – for example, continuously asking their loved one to do something will not result in this happening but increases bad feeling and conflict within the family. Focusing on the development of effective communication therefore can have a beneficial impact on day-to-day life, reducing conflict and stress within the family environment.

Communication styles within families often develop over many years and it may be difficult to introduce positive changes to this. The family members should be encouraged to practise each skill, both in and between sessions, so that they become more comfortable with them. Introducing the skill of expressing pleasant feelings to one another is one of the first components of communication training for family members. By acknowledging when someone does something that pleases others, they are more likely to repeat the behaviour, while feeling appreciated and valued in doing so.

Expressing pleasant feelings

> *Mental health nurse:* How would it help you as a family if others took time to comment and show their appreciation when someone does something positive for somebody else?

Allow all family members to comment.

> *Mental health nurse:* Acknowledging when others do something that pleases us can encourage them to continue doing so and lets them know that they are appreciated for their efforts. It can also help to create an atmosphere where family members can work together, and helps reduce criticism and confrontation. I would like to introduce a skill of expressing pleasant feelings within the family unit. Can you think of a recent example when somebody within the family did something that pleased you?

Use the family's specific example to role-play the skill. For example:

> *Family member Joan:* Yes, Peter cleaned the kitchen at the weekend, which saved me having to do it when I came home from work.
> *Mental health nurse:* That's great. What did you say to Peter when he cleaned the kitchen?
> *Family member Joan:* I don't think I said anything. I was just relieved that it was one less thing for me to do after a really busy day.
> *Mental health nurse:* If we use this example to role-play expressing pleasant feelings, I would like you to look at Peter and tell him exactly what he did that pleased you and how it made you feel. I would like all other family members to observe and comment at the end on what they observed.
> *Family member Joan:* [to Peter] Peter, thank you for cleaning the kitchen for me at the weekend, especially the oven. I was so relieved and very pleased that it was one less job for me to do when I got home. I really appreciated it.
> *Mental health nurse:* [to other family members] What did you like about the way Joan spoke to Peter?

Again, get all family members to give positive feedback.

> *Family member Alan:* I liked the way Joan said she really appreciated that Peter had cleaned the kitchen, especially the oven as it is the job she complains about the most.
>
> *Family member Paul:* I liked the way that Joan spoke, she sounded as though she really meant it.
>
> *Mental health nurse:* Thank you Alan and Paul. Is there anything that Joan could have done differently when she spoke to Peter?
>
> *Family member Alan:* Well, she didn't really look at Peter when she spoke to him, perhaps she did briefly but then she looked at the floor.
>
> *Mental health nurse:* Joan, let's practise that again, but this time I would really like you to face Peter and look at him when you talk.

Making a positive request

By asking others to do something to work out a problem in a positive way, issues are often resolved before the situation escalates into a greater problem. Introducing the skill of making a positive request can therefore help family members address issues as they arise, reducing the overall stress that can be experienced when they are left unresolved.

> *Mental health nurse:* Continuing with our work on communication skills, I would now like us to focus on making a positive request. How would it help you as a family if you were able to ask for things in a positive way?

Allow all family members to comment.

> *MN nurse:* Sometimes we want other family members to do something or change the way in which they do something. Often when we think we are asking them to do this it can lead to tension as the other person can view it as being demanding or nagging. Asking others to do something in a more positive and constructive way can create a more harmonious environment and they are more likely to do the task. Can you think of a recent example when someone asked you to do something?
>
> *Family member Peter:* Mum always gets on at me to tidy my room, but I like it the way it is. She is always having a go.
>
> *Family member Joan:* Alan asked me this morning to go to the post office for him.
>
> *Family member Alan:* Paul gets on to me about the mess I make in the bathroom. He's always going on at me to clean up, but we usually end up in an argument.
>
> *Mental health nurse:* Thank you, you have all given some very good examples. Perhaps if we use the example that Alan has given we can practise

the skill of making a positive request. Paul, I would like you to look at Alan and tell him exactly what you would like him to do and how it would make you feel if he did it. I would like all other family members to observe and comment at the end on what they observed.

Family member Paul: Alan, I would like you to clean and tidy the bathroom after you have used it. It would make me very happy and be one less thing for me to do when I come home from work.

Mental health nurse: [to other family members] What did you like about the way Paul spoke to Alan?

Family member Joan: I liked the way Paul looked at Alan when he spoke.

Family member Peter: I liked the way Paul told Alan how it would make him feel if he tidied the bathroom. It showed Alan that his actions were having an impact on Paul after coming in from work.

Mental health nurse: Thank you Joan and Peter. Is there anything that Paul could have done differently when he spoke to Alan?

Expressing unpleasant feelings

Just as important as expressing pleasant feelings, family members should be encouraged to express unpleasant feelings in a positive and constructive manner. In doing so, conflict within the family can be reduced as, again, issues are dealt with as they arise.

Mental health nurse: How would it help you as a family if you were able to say things to one another you find difficult or upsetting?

Allow all family members to comment.

Mental health nurse: When others do something that upsets us it can be helpful to discuss this by describing the situation, and stating what specifically is upsetting you and how it makes you feel. Using the skills learned earlier, making a positive request offering an alternative solution can positively impact on the situation. This, again, can help to create an atmosphere where family members can work together and avoid situations escalating, helping to reduce criticism and tension. I would like to introduce the skill of expressing unpleasant feelings within the family unit. Can you think of a recent example when something happened within the family and you found it difficult to say how you felt?

Use the family's specific example to role-play the skill. For example:

Family member Joan: Yes, Alan didn't put the rubbish out on Tuesday so we now have to wait until the next bin collection in two weeks' time.

Mental health nurse: If we use this example to role-play expressing unpleasant feelings, I would like you to look at Alan and tell him exactly what he did that upset you and how it made you feel. I would then like you to make a positive request to Alan to try to resolve the issue that is causing you to have these feelings. I would like all other family members to observe and comment at the end on what they observed.

Family member Joan: [*to Alan*] Alan, when you didn't put the rubbish out this week it made me feel really angry and upset. I would appreciate it if you could remember to put the rubbish out, it would mean a lot to me.

Mental health nurse: Thank you Joan. [*to other family members*] What did Joan do well when talking to Alan?

Family member Peter: I liked the way Joan was able to say that she was upset about the bins. She didn't raise her voice or become argumentative, but stated how it made her feel.

Family member Paul: I liked the way that Joan made a positive request. It somehow didn't sound so negative.

Mental health nurse: Is there anything that Joan could have done differently when she spoke to Alan?

Family member Paul: Although Joan stated how it made her feel when Alan didn't put the bins out, she could have said how it would make her feel if he put them out next time. Joan said it would mean a lot to her but didn't state a specific feeling.

Mental health nurse: Joan, lets practise that again, but this time I would really like you to say how it would make you feel if Alan puts the rubbish out next time.

Box 16.3 contains a third learning opportunity.

Box 16.3 Activity opportunity

Consider how practising the different components of communication skills may feel as a family member within the family session. What are the advantages and disadvantages in asking family members to role-play specific scenarios that have recently occurred within the family? How would you respond if the family chose difficult situations that could lead to hostility or criticism? What if the family stated they felt silly and self-conscious in the role play, or that it felt artificial – how would you respond?

Problem solving

Effective communication is the foundation of effective problem solving within the family. Following the information gained from the individual family assessment, the nurse will have an understanding of how issues are resolved within the family. It is important to recognise strengths within the family, and to acknowledge and build on these. A six-step method is used within the family sessions, which requires the family to work collaboratively in identifying problems and goals, discussing and choosing possible solutions and developing a plan together to implement the best solution. Problem solving is discussed in more depth in Chapter 4.

Six-step approach to problem solving:

1. define the problem (or goal)

2. list all possible solutions

3. discuss each possible solution

4. choose the best solution

5. plan how to carry out the best solution

6. review results.

Homework

It is important to emphasise from the start the importance of practising each skill between sessions. Introducing the idea of a family meeting between sessions is a useful way of ensuring the family set time aside each week to meet and discuss their goals and problems. The more families practise the specific skills the more comfortable they will become using them until they become second nature. It is important that the mental health nurse asks family members how the homework has gone between sessions, and allows family members to feed back, giving positive feedback and encouragement.

Conclusion

The aim of this chapter has been to introduce family intervention as a therapeutic intervention for those with psychosis, their families and carers. Its value and use in mental health nursing has been explored, and the use of specific skills in relation to expressing pleasant feelings, making positive requests and expressing unpleasant feelings has been outlined.

It should now be clear that family intervention should be offered to all those who experience psychosis, forming an essential component of the care and treatment of the client group. When working with families, the building of a therapeutic relationship with each family member is just as important as the relationship between the mental health nurse and the individual client. Working collaboratively with all family members, conducting individual family member assessments and focusing on the development of effective communication skills can all have a beneficial impact on the day-to-day lives of family members, reducing conflict and stress within the family environment.

The mental health nurse should demonstrate high levels of interpersonal skills and be confident in working with groups of people. Furthermore, he or she should be knowledgeable, creative and flexible in their approach with family members. Supervision specific to family intervention should be sought from suitably qualified practitioners to ensure mental health nurses have the opportunity to acknowledge, reflect upon, explore and challenge their practice, as well as to ensure high-quality delivery of the intervention.

Suggested reading

Fadden, G. (2009) Family interventions and psychosis, in Beinart, H., Kennedy, P. and Llewelyn, S. (eds) *Clinical Psychology in Practice*. Oxford: Blackwell Publishing.

This book is aimed at psychologists, but the author is highly regarded in the field and this chapter will appeal to nurses and others with interests in this area.

Kuipers, E., Leff, J. and Lam, D. (2002) *Family Work for Schizophrenia: A Practical Guide*, 2nd edn. London: Gaskell Press.

This relatively short book is aimed at practitioners, including nurses, wanting to incorporate family work into their everyday practice.

References

Bebbington, P. and Kuipers, L. (1994) The predictive utility of expressed emotion in schizophrenia: an aggregate analysis. *Psychological Medicine*, 24, 3, 707–718.

Bradshaw, T., Lovell, K. and Richards, D. (2000) PSI and COPE. *Mental Health Nursing*, 20, 10–14.

Bradshaw, T., Mairs, H. and Lowndes, F. (2003) COPE: a four year progress review. *Mental Health Nursing*, 23, 4–6.

Brown, G., Birley, J. and Wing, J. (1972) The influence of family life on the course of schizophrenic disorders: a replication. *British Journal of Psychiatry*, 121, 241–258.

Brown, G., Carstairs, G. and Topping, G. (1958) Post hospital adjustment of chronic mental patients. *The Lancet*, ii, 685–689.

Doornbos, M. (2002) Family care givers and the mental health care system: reality and dreams. *Archives of Psychiatric Nursing*, 16, 1, 39–46.

Fadden, G. (1998) Research update: psychoeducational family interventions. *Journal of Family Therapy*, 20, 293–309.

Falloon, I.R.H., Boyd, J.L. and McGill, C.W. (1984) *Family Care of Schizophrenia: A Problem-solving Approach to the Treatment of Mental Illness*. New York: Guilford Press.

Gamble, C. (1997) The THORN nursing programme: its past, present and future. *Mental Health Care*, 1, 3, 95–97.

Kavanagh, D. (1992) Recent developments in expressed emotion and schizophrenia. *British Journal of Psychiatry*, 160, 601–620.

Kuipers, E. (2006) Family interventions in schizophrenia: evidence for efficacy and proposed mechanisms for change. *Journal of Family Therapy*, 28, 73–80.

Kuipers, E. and Bebbington, P. (2005) *Research on Burden and Coping Strategies in Families of People with Mental Disorders: Problems and Perspectives.* Chichester: Wiley.

National Institute for Health and Care Excellence (2014) *Psychosis and Schizophrenia in Adults: Treatment and Management.* London: National Institute for Health and Care Excellence.

National Institute for Health and Clinical Excellence (2009) *Schizophrenia: Core Interventions in the Treatment and Management of Schizophrenia in Primary and Secondary Care* (update). London: National Institute for Health and Clinical Excellence.

Nuechterlain, K. and Dawson, M. (1984) A heuristic vulnerability-stress model of schizophrenic episodes. *Schizophrenia Bulletin,* 10, 300–312.

Raune, D., Kuipers, E. and Bebbington, P. (2004) EE at first episode psychosis: investigating a carer appraised model. *British Journal of Psychiatry,* 184, 321–326.

Scazufca, M. and Kuipers, E. (1996) Links between expressed emotion and burden of care in relatives of patients with schizophrenia. *British Journal of Psychiatry,* 168, 580–587.

Thornicroft, G., Tansella, M., Becker, T., Knapp, M., Leese, M., Schene, A. and Vazquez-Barquero, J. (2004) EPSILON study group. The personal impact of schizophrenia in Europe. *Schizophrenia Research,* 69, 125–132.

Vaughn, C. and Leff, J. (1976) The influence of family and social factors on the cause of psychiatric illness: a comparison of schizophrenic and depressed neurotic patients. *British Journal of Psychiatry,* 129, 125–137.

Zubin, J. and Spring, B. (1997) Vulnerability: a new view of schizophrenia. *Journal of Abnormal Psychology,* 86, 103–126.

Index

'5 Ws', assessment interviews 13–15
activities
  assessment interviews 18–19
  family intervention in psychosis 209,
   210, 214
  family therapies 190
  groups 202
  mindfulness 164
  psychoeducation 99
  volatile situations 176
affirmations, person-centred
  counselling 46
algorithmic methods, problem solving
  76
ambivalence, motivational interviewing
  62, 67
assessment
  family intervention in psychosis
   206–9
  problem solving 78–80
assessment interviews 6–19
  '5 Ws' 13–15
  activities 18–19
  areas of assessment 9–10
  care and treatment plans (CTPs) 7
  Care Programme Approach (CPA) 7
  closing the interview 17
  collaborative agenda 12–13
  formulation 15–17
  gathering information 13–15
  mental health assessment 7–8

National Institute for Health and
  Care Excellence (NICE) 8, 9
National Patient Safety Agency
  (NPSA) 9–10
Nursing and Midwifery Council
  (NMC) 6
open questions 13–15
opportunities 8–9
preparation 10–11
relationship building 12–13
SBAR: Situation–Background–
  Assessment–Recommendation 18
sharing information 17–18
SMART goals 16–17
structure 11–12
tools 10–11
values and principles 10
attention, Three Axioms of Mindfulness
  160–1, 162, 163
attitude, Three Axioms of Mindfulness
  160–1

behavioural experiments, unhelpful
  thoughts 111–13
behavioural management 143–52
  see also cognitive behavioural
   therapy (CBT)
  depression and anxiety 144–7
  evaluation 150–1
  evidence-based practice 147
  measuring behaviour 148–9

monitoring behaviour 149
operant conditioning 145–7
reinforcement, positive/negative 146–7
reinforcing desired behaviour 149–50
SMART objectives 149, 150–1
social skills training 151–2
step-by-step guide 147–51
theoretical basis 144–7
below-the-surface processes, supervision 27–9
bipolar disorder (BPD)
psychoeducation 91, 92–3
relapse prevention (RP) 91, 135–6
Self-Management Programme 95
brainstorming, problem solving method 76
British Psychological Society's Division for Clinical Psychology 80

care and treatment plans (CTPs), assessment interviews 7
Care Programme Approach (CPA), assessment interviews 7
CBT see cognitive behavioural therapy
change motivation, motivational interviewing 63–8
change plan, motivational interviewing 68–9
child development, person-centred counselling 36, 37–8
clarifying, person-centred counselling 46
closing the interview, assessment interviews 17
cognition levels 104–5
cognitive behavioural therapy (CBT) 102–15
see also behavioural management
depression and anxiety 103–4
history 103–4
key points 103–6
motivational interviewing 62
unhelpful thoughts 102–15
cognitive restructuring 106
cognitive therapy, vs mindfulness 158
collaborative agenda, assessment interviews 12–13
collaborative style, problem solving 82

communication skills, family intervention in psychosis 210–11
communication styles, motivational interviewing 63–8
confirmation bias, problem solving 84
core beliefs, cognition level 104
core skills
motivational interviewing 63–9
person-centred counselling 42–6
counselling see person-centred counselling
countertransference, supervision 28–9
CPA see Care Programme Approach
CTPs see care and treatment plans
cycle of change, relapse prevention (RP) 131–2

DBT see dialectical behaviour therapy
dementia 117–28
example 119–21
nine-stage model 124
symptoms 121–2
validation approach 117–28
depression and anxiety
behavioural management 144–7
cognitive behavioural therapy (CBT) 103–4
relapse prevention (RP) 134–40
dialectical behaviour therapy (DBT), mindfulness 159
discrepancy development, motivational interviewing 63
dynamic clinical variables, volatile situations 169
dysfunctional assumptions, cognition level 104

empathic reflecting, person-centred counselling 46
empathy
motivational interviewing 63
person-centred counselling 41–2
supervision 28–9
End of Life Namaste Care Program 127
European Brief Therapy Association, solution-focused therapy 58
evidence, problem solving 82–3
evidence base
mindfulness 159

Mindfulness Based Stress Reduction (MBSR) 159
evidence-based practice
  behavioural management 147
  psychoeducation 90–1
expressing pleasant feelings, family intervention in psychosis 211–12
expressing unpleasant feelings, family intervention in psychosis 213–14

family intervention in psychosis 204–16
  activities 209, 210, 214
  assessment 206–9
  Behavioural Family Therapy 206
  communication skills 210–11
  COPE programme 206
  engagement 206–9
  expressing pleasant feelings 211–12
  expressing unpleasant feelings 213–14
  homework 215
  National Institute for Health and Care Excellence (NICE) 205, 206
  parts 208
  positive requests 212
  problem solving 214–15
  psychoeducation 209–10
  Schizophrenia Commission 206
  theoretical basis 205–6
  Thorn course 206
family therapies 181–90
  activities 190
  assessment and formulation 183
  externalisation of the problem 184–9
  genograms 183
  Improving Access to Psychological Therapies programme 182
  mapping the relational context 183
  questions as a starting point 183–4
  theoretical basis 182
fear, overcoming 144
formulation, assessment interviews 15–17

gathering information, assessment interviews 13–15
goal setting, motivational interviewing 68–9
groups 192–202
  action phase 194, 196
  activities 202
  adjourning phase 201
  closed groups 194
  cohesion 198
  constraints 195
  cooperation 197
  evaluation 201–2
  facilitating groups 195–202
  forming stage 197–9
  ground rules 198
  group process 194–5, 197–202
  leadership style 196–7
  norming phase 201
  open groups 194
  orientation phase 194, 196
  performing phase 201
  planning 195–6
  pre-discharge group 198–9, 200
  preparing 195–6
  record keeping 201–2
  social-interactional support 198
  storming phase 199–200
  structured groups 193
  supportive groups 194
  termination phase 194, 196, 201
  therapeutic groups 193
  types of group 193–4
  unstructured groups 193–4
GROW (Goal, Reality, Options and Way forward), problem solving 81–2
guided discovery, unhelpful thoughts 106, 108–10

heuristic methods, problem solving 76
human potential, person-centred counselling 36–7
humanistic psychology, person-centred counselling 36

ICS see interacting cognitive subsystems
identity, maintaining, validation approach 121–2, 125
intention, Three Axioms of Mindfulness 160–1, 163
interacting cognitive subsystems (ICS), mindfulness 156–7
interviews see assessment interviews; motivational interviewing

lateral thinking, problem solving 82
listening skills, person-centred
    counselling 42–6

Manchester Care Assessment Schedule
    (MANCAS), problem assessment
    79
MBCT *see* Mindfulness Based Cognitive
    Therapy
MBSR *see* Mindfulness Based Stress
    Reduction
mental health assessment, assessment
    interviews 7–8
mental health nursing
    motivational interviewing 63
    supervision 21–2
mindfulness 154–64
    activities 164
    appropriate use 155–6
    background 156
    dialectical behaviour therapy (DBT)
        159
    evidence base 159
    interacting cognitive subsystems
        (ICS) 156–7
    Mindfulness Based Cognitive
        Therapy (MBCT) 155–6
    Mindfulness Based Stress Reduction
        (MBSR) 155–6
    mindfulness practice 159–63
    reflection 161–2
    safe use 155–6
    theoretical basis 155–7
    therapeutic benefits 157–8
    Three Axioms of Mindfulness 160–1
    vs cognitive therapy 158
Mindfulness Based Cognitive Therapy
    (MBCT) 155–6
Mindfulness Based Stress Reduction
    (MBSR) 155–6
mind-mapping, problem solving 82
minimal prompts, person-centred
    counselling 45–6
motivational interviewing 60–71
    see also person-centred
        counselling
    agenda mapping 65
    ambivalence 62, 67

change motivation 63–8
change plan 68–9
cognitive behavioural therapy (CBT)
    62
communication styles 63–8
core skills 63–9
decisional balance 67–8
defining 61
discrepancy development 63
empathy 63
features 62–3, 69
goal setting 68–9
key principles 63–8
mental health nursing 63
planning 68–9
rapport 63–8
relational component 61
resistance 63
self-efficacy 63
technical component 61

National Institute for Health and Care
    Excellence (NICE)
    assessment interviews 8, 9
    family intervention in psychosis 205,
        206
    psychoeducation 88, 89
    relapse prevention (RP) 133
    schizophrenia 206
    volatile situations 167
National Patient Safety Agency (NPSA),
    assessment interviews 9–10
NATs *see* negative automatic thoughts
needs, feelings and emotions, validation
    approach 121–2
negative automatic thoughts (NATs)
    102–15
    see also unhelpful thoughts
    cognition level 104
    problems 110–11
NICE *see* National Institute for Health
    and Care Excellence
nine-stage model, dementia 124
NMC *see* Nursing and Midwifery
    Council
NPSA *see* National Patient Safety Agency
Nursing and Midwifery Council (NMC)
    assessment interviews 6

requirements 6, 12, 18, 167–8
validation approach 118
volatile situations 167–8
nursing process, problem solving
method 77–8

open questions
assessment interviews 13–15
person-centred counselling 45
operant conditioning, behavioural
management 145–7
Orem's Self Care Model, problem
assessment 79

parallel processes, supervision 28–9
paraphrasing, person-centred
counselling 46
PDCA (Plan– Do–Check–Act), problem
solving method 76–7
person-centred counselling 35–47
see also motivational interviewing
child development 36, 37–8
core skills 42–6
criticism 47
empathy 41–2
human potential 36–7
humanistic psychology 36
integrating qualities and skills 39–42
listening skills 42–6
rapport 41–2
relationships 37
responding skills 42–6
self/self-awareness 37–9
structuring time and support 40
therapeutic relationship 37
therapeutic sessions 39–42
unconditional positive regard 37–8
personhood, maintaining, validation
approach 122, 124–5
planning
motivational interviewing 68–9
problem solving 81–3
Positive Person Work, validation
approach 123–4
positive requests, family intervention in
psychosis 212
preparation, assessment interviews
10–11

problem solving 74–86
algorithmic methods 76
assessment 78–80
brainstorming 76
collaborative style 82
confirmation bias 84
crystallising the problem 80
defining 'problem' 75
evaluation 84
evidence 82–3
family intervention in psychosis
214–15
GROW (Goal, Reality, Options and
Way forward) 81–2
heuristic methods 76
identifying the problem 78–80
implementation 83
lateral thinking 82
Manchester Care Assessment
Schedule (MANCAS) 79
mind-mapping 82
nursing process 77–8
Orem's Self Care Model 79
PDCA (Plan– Do–Check–Act) 76–7
planning 81–3
problem identification 79–80
reassessment 84
reflection 85
risk assessment 79–80
Shewhart Cycle 76–7
six-step approach 215
SMART goals 81–2
solution failure 85–6
Structured Clinical Interview for
DSM-IV (SCID) 79
testing solutions 83
theoretical basis 75–6
Tidal Model 79
trial-and-error methods 75
projective identification, supervision
28–9
psychoeducation 88–99
activities 99
bipolar disorder (BPD) 91, 92–3
defining 88
evidence-based practice 90–1
family intervention in psychosis
209–10

group sessions 92–8
leaders 95
National Institute for Health and
      Care Excellence (NICE) 88, 89
participants 95–6
programmes 92–5
service user involvement 95
theoretical background 89–90
therapeutic approach 91–2
thought records/diaries 108
psychosis, family intervention *see*
      family intervention in psychosis

rapport
      motivational interviewing 63–8
      person-centred counselling 41–2
reflecting key words, person-centred
      counselling 46
reflection
      empathic reflecting, person-centred
            counselling 46
      mindfulness 161–2
      problem solving 85
      supervision 26
reinforcement, positive/negative,
      behavioural management 146–7
relapse prevention (RP) 130–41
      assess stage 137–8
      bipolar disorder (BPD) 91, 135–6
      case study 134–40
      cycle of change 131–2
      depression and anxiety 134–40
      educate stage 135–7
      flexibility 133
      guiding principles 134–5
      implement stage 139
      key stages 135–9
      National Institute for Health and
            Care Excellence (NICE) 133
      plan stage 138–9
      practice skills 134–40
      stress-vulnerability model 132–3,
            135–6
      theoretical background 131–3
relationship building, assessment
      interviews 12–13
relationships
      person-centred counselling 37

supervision 24–5, 27–9
      therapeutic relationship 37
reminiscence, validation approach 125–6
resistance, motivational interviewing
      63
responding skills, person-centred
      counselling 42–6
risk assessment, problem solving 79–80
RP *see* relapse prevention

SBAR: Situation–Background–
      Assessment–Recommendation,
      assessment interviews 18
schizophrenia
      see also family intervention in
            psychosis
      National Institute for Health and
            Care Excellence (NICE) 206
Schizophrenia Commission, family
      intervention in psychosis 206
SCID *see* Structured Clinical Interview
      for DSM-IV
self-disclosure, person-centred
      counselling 46
self-efficacy, motivational interviewing
      63
Self-Management Programme, bipolar
      disorder (BPD) 95
self/self-awareness, person-centred
      counselling 37–9
sharing information, assessment
      interviews 17–18
Shewhart Cycle, problem solving
      method 76–7
six-step approach, problem solving 215
SMART goals
      assessment interviews 16–17
      problem solving 81–2
SMART objectives, behavioural
      management 149, 150–1
social skills training, behavioural
      management 151–2
Socratic dialogue, unhelpful thoughts
      106, 108–10
solution-focused therapy 49–58
      assumptions 50–1, 52
      European Brief Therapy Association
            58

feedback 56–7
limitations 50–1
locating exceptions 56
miracle questions 54–5
problem identification 53–4
scaling questions 55
skills development 52–7
solution amplification 54–6
steps 52–7
theoretical basis 50–1
using/uses 49, 51
Sonas aPc (Activating the Potential to Communicate), validation approach 127
stress-vulnerability model, relapse prevention (RP) 132–3, 135–6
structure, assessment interviews 11–12
Structured Clinical Interview for DSM-IV (SCID), problem assessment 79
summarising, person-centred counselling 46
supervision 21–30
below-the-surface processes 27–9
continuity over time 25–6
countertransference 28–9
effectiveness 23
elements 25–6
emotions 27
empathy 28–9
functions 22
learning 27
mental health nursing 21–2
models 29
monitoring 27
parallel processes 28–9
practicalities 29
projective identification 28–9
questions 29–30
reasons for 22–3
reflection 26
relationships 24–5, 27–9
supervisee 24–5
supervisor's role 24
therapy 24–5
symptoms of dementia 121–2

therapeutic relationship, person-centred counselling 37

therapeutic silence, person-centred counselling 46
therapy, supervision 24–5
thinking errors
problems 110–11
unhelpful thoughts 104–5, 110–11
thought records/diaries, unhelpful thoughts 107–8
Three Axioms of Mindfulness 160–1
Tidal Model, problem assessment 79
tools, assessment interviews 10–11
trial-and-error methods, problem solving 75

unhelpful thoughts
see also negative automatic thoughts (NATs)
behavioural experiments 111–13
cognitive behavioural therapy (CBT) 102–15
cognitive restructuring 106
guided discovery 106, 108–10
Socratic dialogue 106, 108–10
thinking errors 104–5, 110–11
thought records/diaries 107–8

validation approach 117–28
assumptions 119
defining 'validation therapy' 118–19
dementia 117–28
End of Life Namaste Care Program 127
example 119–21
Identity, maintaining 121–2, 125
needs, feelings and emotions 121–2
Nursing and Midwifery Council (NMC) 118
personhood, maintaining 122, 124–5
Positive Person Work 123–4
principles 118–19
reminiscence 125–6
sensory approaches 126
skills 118, 122–3
Sonas aPc (Activating the Potential to Communicate) 127
symptoms of dementia 121–2
values and principles, assessment interviews 10

verbal aggression, volatile situations
169
verbal communication, volatile
situations 170
volatile situations 167–76
activities 176
dynamic clinical variables 169
historical factors 168

important points 175
National Institute for Health and
Care Excellence (NICE) 167
Nursing and Midwifery Council
(NMC) 167–8
theoretical basis 168–9
verbal aggression 169
verbal communication 170

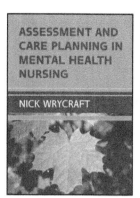

Assessment and Care Planning in Mental Health
Nursing

Nick Wrycraft

ISBN: 9780335262984 (Paperback)
eBook: 9780335262991
2015

Assessment of mental health problems is a challenging area of practice that
covers a range of symptoms and behaviours – and involves building a
trusting relationship with the service user while also using specialist skills.
Care planning involves translating information emerging from assessment to
collaboratively identify goals and aspirations that are meaningful yet also
realistic and personalized.

The first section of the book explores core aspects of assessment including
communication skills and engaging the service user before considering risk
assessment, care planning, interventions, relapse prevention and reflection.
The next section will be ideal for quick reference during practice and looks
at 23 different clinical behaviours that nurses will assess, under 4 categories:

> Physical factors in mental health
> Behavioural aspects in mental health
> The role of thoughts in mental health
> Feelings in mental health

www.mheducation.co.uk

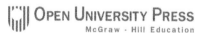

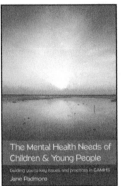

The Mental Health Needs of Children and Young People
Guiding you to key issues and practices in CAMHS

Padmore

ISBN: 9780335263905 (Paperback)
eBook: 9780335263912
2015

This book is an accessible and practical guide to all of the key issues and practices in mental health care for children and young people, aimed at all health and social care professionals working with this age group and partner agencies who work alongside child and adolescent mental health services.

Written by an expert in the field, the book brings clarity to practice by exploring and explaining the context, role and processes involving child and adolescent mental health services. It also sets out the specific mental health difficulties young people and their families present to services as well as how to make good health assessments, plans and interventions used in the treatment of children and young people – including managing risk and safeguarding.

Key features include:

> Questions to encourage your reflection on different key issues in your own practice
> Up-to-date information on current policy
> Key points summaries and suggested further reading at the end of each chapter

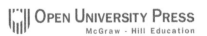

www.mheducation.co.uk

OPEN UNIVERSITY PRESS
McGraw - Hill Education

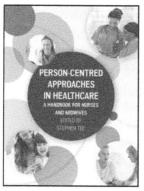

Person-centred approaches in healthcare
A handbook for nurses and midwives

Stephen Tee

ISBN: 9780335263585 (Paperback)
eBook: 9780335263592
2016

Written by practitioners, academics and, more importantly, the people who use health services, this unique text examines the application of person-centred principles across a range of healthcare contexts. It will provide you with the essential skills, techniques and strategies needed to deliver person-centred care.

Patients and service users should be at the heart of healthcare delivery and this book will equip nurses and midwives by connecting the reader to the lived experience of those receiving healthcare. It examines issues across the lifespan and reveals how person-centred care can best be achieved by working in partnership.

Key areas include:

Maternity care
Family care including health visiting
Adolescent care
Adult critical care
Diseases including diabetes and arthritis
Care for people with long term mental health problems
Intellectual disabilities
Care of carers

www.mheducation.co.uk

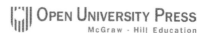

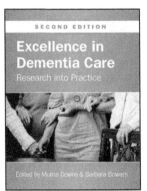

Excellence in Dementia Care
Principles and Practices
Second Edition

Downs and Bowers

ISBN: 9780335245338 (Paperback)
eBook: 9780335245345
2014

This scholarly yet accessible textbook is the most comprehensive single text in the field of dementia care. Drawn from research evidence, international expertise and good practice guidelines, the book has been crafted alongside people with dementia and their families. Case studies and quotes in every chapter illustrate the realities of living with dementia and bring the theory to life.

Key topics include:

- Dementia friendly communities
- Representations of dementia in the media
- Younger people with dementia
- The arts and dementia
- Whole person assessment
- Dementia friendly physical design
- Transitions in care
- Enhancing relationships between families and those with dementia

www.openup.co.uk

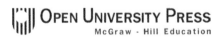

OPEN UNIVERSITY PRESS
McGraw - Hill Education